STRESS-ADDICTION

A new Theory on Evolution

*To Lorica
with love
Branko
Sredor, July 89*

Branko Bokun

STRESS-ADDICTION
A new Theory on Evolution

Vita Books
26 Chelsea Square
London SW3

© Branko Bokun 1989

'First published in 1989 by
Vita Books
26 Chelsea Square, London SW3

ISBN 0 9510525 3 5

1. Anthropology   2. Sociology
3. Psychiatry   4. Economics

All rights reserved.
No parts of this book may be reproduced without permission from the publisher, except for quotation of brief passages in criticism.

Printed in Great Britain by
Biddles Ltd., Guildford and Kings Lynn.

Contents

Introduction	1
Origin of life	9
The cell	13
First Organism	16
Reproduction of life	19
Morphogenesis	22
Genes	24
Evolution	33
Evolution of humans	37
Anxiety	46
Anxiety and the span of life	56
Anxiety and growth	59
Stress	67
Fatigue	86
Pain	91
Stress-addiction	93
Individuality	98
Courses in anxiety and stress	136

My grateful thanks to Anne Loudon for her help in writing this book, and also to Misha Lukic for his valuable advice.

Introduction

I think that we would be in a better position to understand fears and anxieties if we discovered their real essences. We could only do that if we guessed their origins correctly. In order to do this we should try to penetrate into the very heart of living matter, of life itself.

The origin of life has intrigued the human mind ever since it started.

At the outset of the mind's activity, mythology tried to placate human curiosity, to place man in the universe.

Many people still believe in the Bible's explanation, that the omnipotent God created everything from nothing in six days. Some even believe that God completed His creation on Sunday, the 23rd October 4.004BC.

There are those who claim that the first organic compounds were brought to our planet from space.

If life brought from space could have prospered on Earth's environment, surely that same environment would have been capable of creating that life.

For most scientists today, a random shuffling of inorganic molecules in the primeval soup, some 3,500 million years ago, produced the first organic molecules. The rest was evolution based mainly on genetic mutation followed by natural selection and the survival of the fittest.

Life is an order which evolved from the order of matter, like the order of matter evolved from that of energy, like the order of energy evolved from the order which preceded it, and which is beyond our comprehension. Even further beyond our comprehension are orders that preceded the one from which the order of energy evolved.

Any new order must have started with an increase in the instability of the previous order, or in a part of it.

Many insist that before the appearance of our universe of matter there was a stability or a symmetry between the matter and anti-matter particles.

If this was true we would not be here, as the universe of matter would have never evolved from stability. Nothing happens in stability or symmetry, as they imply non-existence, they imply immobility.

Whatever exists must be active. An activity can only be triggered off and carried on by instability. Existence consists of instability. Even the level of an existence is related to its level of instability.

What could the activity of an instability be?

Instability can only have one activity: the pursuit of lesser instability.

In fact, the supreme law ruling the universe and everything that exists in it is, in my view, the tendency towards a lesser instability. Becoming implies instability.

What we call 'fundamental forces' operating in the universe (gravity, electro-magnetism, strong and weak nuclear forces) could be considered as the consequences of the universal law of instability striving towards a lesser instability.

The beginning of any new order or of any new existence must be preceded by a mutation in the instability of the previous order or a previous existence.

Only a mutation which is increasing the instability in an order or an existence can evolve towards a new order or a new existence. Only an increased instability can jump into a novelty in evolution.

Being the product of an increase in instability, a novelty in evolution brings an increase in the complexity which implies an increase in instability and vulnerability.

INTRODUCTION

Instability tends to find its lesser instability through expansion. Through expansion, instability ends in over-expansion, followed by breakdown, resulting in the lesser instability of the previous existence.

In the universe, contraction finds its initial push in over-expansion. The new expansion finds its initial propulsion in over-contraction.

In the relationship or pairing between matter and anti-matter particles, there must have been, however minimal, an instability, an asymmetry.

In this instability some matter particles must have undergone a mutation in their instability, increasing it, and this must have been the reason for their escape into a new order.

Many insist that the universe of anti-matter should be a mirror image of our universe of matter.

If the universe of anti-matter ever existed it would be a different universe, it would be less unstable than that of matter.

The minimal instability reached by an existence is its dormant state. Some existence can remain dormant for billions of years, some a few seconds.

The irritation of a dormant state can revive an existence.

By increasing instability, a strong or persevering irritation can also create a mutation in the instability of an existence from which a new existence can evolve.

Any further reduction of the instability, however, beyond the dormant state of an existence, can bring an end to the existence, it can provoke the jump into the lesser instability of the previous existence, of the previous order. Each existence craves for the lesser instability of the previous existence.

In human terms one could venture that the general feeling of everything in the universe is that of nostalgia, of a desire to return to the lost paradise of the previous existence. Everything that exists must carry a memory of its past existences.

Each new order appears smaller than the previous one from which it evolved. The world of matter compared to that of energy is very small, the living world compared to that of matter is even smaller, so is the world of multicellular organisms compared to that of bacteria from which it evolved.

Each new order seems to become more complex and more unstable. In fact, the only difference between the order of inorganic matter and the order of organic matter is that the latter is more unstable than the former. It is, in fact, this extra instability that provides the living world with what we call life's energy.

It is this increased instability that provided and continued to provide the main characteristics of organic order: flexibility, sensibility, perceptibility and adaptability. The greater the instability of an organism or of a species, the more prominent these characteristics are.

It is in this high instability of organic order that we find the reason for such a variety of forms of life.

Instability, which in organic order reaches precariousness, increases the intensity of the basic drive of the universe: the drive towards a lesser instability.

Any activity of living matter is caused and perpetuated by biochemical precariousness or discomfort in search of a lesser precariousness or a lesser discomfort.

In their search for lesser instability, organisms developed two main drives: the absorbtion of whatever could reduce this discomfort, and the rejection of whatever could increase it. It is the drive for absorbtion of whatever could lessen biochemical instability that helped organisms to develop their taste and distaste. It is the need of biochemical instability for lesser biochemical instability or discomfort that helped organisms to develop their senses and their sensual organs.

Any new order or any new existence increases the instability of all existing orders or existences, because in the universe everything is related to everything else.

The universe and everything in it all follow the same pattern. Everything has its own big bang, its own burst or birth, its own expansion or growth, its own maturity, its own contraction or decay, in order to jump to a new big bang, a new burst or birth, a new expansion or growth, and so on.

In our yo-yo universe everything is cyclical. Some cycles like those between big bangs can last billions of years, some such as human life can last around seventy years, and some like those between heart beats can last less than a second.

In our yo-yo universe, each jump, be it that of an electron jumping from one orbit to another, or the jump of a heart from expansion to contraction, or vice versa, brings an existence to its minimal instability, an instability of the previous existence from which it evolved. For example, with every heart-beat, death occurs for an instant.

In our yo-yo universe, everything has its own expansion and contraction, its own growth and decline.

Expansion and contraction have their own characteristics which are best reflected in living order, and particularly in the animal world and humans.

Increasing instability, expansion is a tense state of existence which makes individuals more selfish, more intolerant and more aggressive.

On the other hand, however, contraction provides radiation. This radiation is reflected in the living world by fruitfulness, fecundity, tolerance and sacrifice.

The characteristics of contraction are present in a latent state in each expansion, and vice versa.

In the animal and human world it seems that contraction's characteristics are more pronounced in females while those of expansion in males.

Science is trying to unveil the secrets of the universe by discovering never-ending subatomic particles. In my view, we might unearth more about the universe and its main law by also analysing the human mind, this latest appearance in its evolution.

By the mind I mean the brain's creation of wishful beliefs, illusions, or hopeful speculations. Our brain's wishful thinking must be the product of the brain's cells which are made up of organelles and particles in a state of instability, in a state of biochemical discomfort.

In fact, our wishful thinking is the reflection of the tendency of our brain's cells and their organisation towards a state of a lesser instability, a lesser biochemical discomfort. However abstract an idea might be, it must have its biochemical origin, it must be a reflection of the biochemical conditions of the brain's cells and their organisation. As any new phenomenon in evolution, the mind must have unfolded from a previous state of instability.

The unpredictability of the brain's cells' instability could be seen in the mind's passions for divinations. Astrology started and evolved with the human mind.

The instability of our brain cells and of the particles composing them is also illustrated in our more or less constant curiosity. In fact, an increase in instability can easily increase curiosity.

Beliefs in order-giving omnipotent gods must be products of the mind's wishful thinking aiming at the placation of the mind's instability and discontent.

With the exception of their dormant states of reduced instability, the brain's cells are more or less in constant restlessness or agitation which produces the mind's discontent with its own restlessness and agitation. This can be seen in the continuous changes in humanity's beliefs and in its moral, political, economic or aesthetic ideas.

The human mind's constant desire to master nature and the universe must have been inspired by the mind's inherent discontent, carried by the biochemical instability of the human brain's cells.

It is in this discontent that our mind's wishful thinking created belief in miracles and the super-natural.

The human mind invented the wishful belief that after death the believer would go to a 'heaven'. The heavens of most beliefs represent stability and harmony, a static state, more in tune with the lesser instability and the lesser agitation of the inorganic matter from which the organic matter evolved.

The idea of death as a liberation must have been inspired by the nostalgia of the brain's cells' molecules for their previous existence.

I feel sure that if a stone was able to produce its own wishful thinking, it would also invent its aspiration of becoming part of its own paradise, which would be a field of energy. A particle must crave to become a wave.

Some people try to escape life and its reality into a state of nirvana or ecstasy, the nearest that the human mind can approach the previous order of inorganic matter, an order of lesser instability and lesser sensitivity.

Modern physics leans on the principle of uncertainty. This idea could only have been discovered by a brain which cells and cells' organisation were in a state of constant instability. In this uncertainty, however, there is one certainty: the tendency of uncertainty towards a lesser uncertainty.

C. G. Jung's archetypes, which were a kind of inherited ideas or belief, supposed to be present in the roots of our species subconsciousness, must, in reality, be a product of human wishful thinking inspired by the biochemical instability of the brain's cells, an instability peculiar to the human species in search of lesser instability.

If the first molecule of living matter had been able to express itself in human terms, it would have stressed that it was in an agitated state, that life was fear. In biblical terms, it could be said: 'At the beginning there was fear, and fear begat life.'

A state of instability is, in fact, a state of fear, a state of suffering. Each organism is used to a certain range of instability. In this range of instability an organism does not notice its fears. We call fears those sensations of biochemical instabilities which are above the usual or normal range.

Fears can also increase with the development of the perceptivity of the brain's cells of their own instabilities. By improving the perceptivity of the brain, evolution merely serves to increase fears and sufferings.

That life consists of fears and sufferings can be deduced, in a certain sense, by near-death experiences. Most of these experiences consist of a sensation of floating in a state of tranquility in a dark tunnel, more in tune with a state of inorganic order than with that of living matter. A sudden appearance of sun-light, the reason for life on earth, brings revival. With revival, the sensation of tension and fear is rewakened.

Origins of life

The main factors contributing to the appearance of the order of life must have been the mild range of the sun's energy, and the frequent daily and seasonal changes in certain regions of our planet. When life started, some 3.5 billion years ago, the days and nights must have been much shorter, as it has been calculated that some 600 million years ago a year on our planet was 424 days.

Temperature played a major role in the formation of inorganic matter. The cooling down of the universe, after the last big bang, forced the components of the neutrons and protons to find a lesser instability in forming these subnuclear particles. At a further decrease of the temperature, the neutrons and protons found a lesser instability by associating in the more complex nuclei. At a further decrease of the cosmic temperature, nuclei and electrons found their lesser instability in forming atoms, which found their lesser instability in forming molecules of matter.

The earth's spring-time conditions must have loosened electrons and their peripheral orbits around atoms of a group of elements, making them more unstable, more excited and more restless. The most exposed elements to these changes must have been carbon hydrogen, nitrogen and oxygen. Atoms of these elements are sensitive to temperature and to its range of changes.

The atoms of living matter are in fact those of inorganic matter in a more unstable, a more agitated state of existence. In its essence, a carbon atom of organic matter is identical to the carbon atom of inorganic matter: they are merely in different states of existence, in different states of instability.

Forced by the increased instability of their electrons and by the greater flexibility of their peripheral orbits, the atoms of the more sensitive elements increased their mutual attraction aiming at a lesser instability by forming associations or aggregations. In search of a lesser instability, these agitated atoms assembled into loosely bonded molecules.

Due to the loose bondage of their components, these molecules developed their own instability which created their tendency towards a lesser instability by forming with other unstable molecules assemblies or macromolecules. These macromolecules are typical of living order.

Consisting of loosely associated molecules, the macromolecules or compounds of the organic matter developed their own instability, their own precariousness, their own vulnerability, which they tried to lessen by becoming part of bigger structures.

This inherent drive of living matter to try to reduce its instability by becoming part of more complex structures opened the way to the formation of the cells, organisms, groups, colonies, States and Empires.

By carrying an increase in needs and demands, any more complex living structure, however, aquires an increase in instability and vulnerability, so, therefore, an increase in its urgency towards a lesser instability. As living matter tries to lessen its instability mainly through growth, it ends up by creating an over-growth, resulting in a break-down, followed by decline and fall.

In fact, life consists of the expansion, over-expansion, breaking-down and decline of macromolecules and their structures.

Organic matter found its main characteristics, such as: aliveness, alertness, sensitivity, curiosity, communicability, learning and memory, in its particular instability.

The mild range of sun energy, coupled with frequent and moderate circadian and seasonal changes in certain regions of our planet, extracted from inorganic matter the components of amino acids, of nucleotides, of carbohydrates and of lipids, these essential molecules of life.

The subunits of amino acids found a lesser instability by forming molecules of amino acids. The amino acids found their lesser instability by forming peptide and polipeptide sequences. These sequences found their lesser instability in folding in on themselves into less unstable globular, three dimensional structures of proteins.

The tendency of a multicellular organism today to fold on itself in distress might find its origin in this characteristic of protein molecules.

Out of the many existing amino acids only a specific twenty of them are used by life. Perhaps this is due to the higher instability of these particular twenty. Their higher instability enabled them to be more active and more co-operative with other molecules.

The components of the nucleosides (nitrogenous bases and sugar) found a lesser instability by assembling into the nucleosides. Under particularly stressful and irritating conditions, caused by temperature or ultraviolet light, nucleosides found a lesser instability by associating with phosphates, forming nucleotides. The nucleotides reduced their precariousness by organising themselves into a chain, making nucleic acids. DNA (deoxyribonucleic acid) and RNA (ribonucleic acid) form the second major building block of life.

DNA must have evolved from some more unstable forms of RNA, which existed before DNA, and which helped the replication of life for a long time.

The DNA chain found a lesser instability by twisting around an axe and, with another twisted DNA strand, forming a tightly compact double helix. In fact, nucleic genes are so tightly coiled, so solidly packed together, that only special enzymes or hormones, in specific conditions, can either separate or activate them.

The instability of certain fatty acids, formed by the precariousness of their components, created gregarious lipids, the third major building block of life.

In search of a lesser instability, lipid molecules aggregated in the form of sheets. In search of their lesser instabilities these lipid sheets formed balloon-like vescicles, precursors of cells' membranes.

A particular combination of unstable atoms of carbon, hydrogen and oxygen found a lesser instability by assembling into carbohydrates, the fourth major building block of life.

The synthesis of each of these blocks of life must have been helped by the other blocks. Only a mutual co-operation of all these blocks could have enabled them to evolve and to form the cell. It is, in fact, this co-operation which created life, and which keeps it going. Co-operation is a result of the activities of a group of participants in search of their lesser instabilities.

The first organic molecules must have been formed under a certain layer of water, vital to protect living matter from the lethal ultraviolet radiation.

Billions of years later, only after photosynthesis had created enough oxygen in the oxygen-starved primeval atmosphere, as to create an ozone protective layer above the atmosphere, could life have dared venture out of the water.

The cell

In search of a lesser precariousness, the organic molecules and compounds originated and perpetuated their associations or integrations. This must have created the cell. This unit of life is, in fact, an organisation of a co-operation of the biochemical instabilities of the cell's components. As in the universe, everything in a cell is related and influenced by everything else. Some co-operative smaller cells, like mitochondria, even integrated with bigger cells.

In the organic primeval soup only co-operative molecules and compounds succeeded in surviving and in evolving.

If the Darwinian theory of natural selection through competition was right, the cell would never have been formed and we would not have been here to discuss the idea of 'the survival of the fittest', an idea so dear to those who consider themselves successful.

The quality and rhythm of the organisation of the permanent activity of a cell must be ruled by the cell's most unstable components: its enzymes and its peptides floating in the cell's cytoplasms.

A cell is an organisation, and an organisation is based on communications, and communications are mainly influenced by the most unstable parts of the organisation, simply because these are the most alert, the most sensitive and the most active.

Being the most vulnerable, therefore the most alert and the most sensitive, these enzymes and these peptides are also an essential factor in the relationship and communication of the cell with its environment.

Sensitivity and perceptivity of the cell's perceptors are under the control of enzymes and peptides.

Being proteins, therefore flexible, enzymes and peptides are also essential factors of the cell's adaptation to its environment.

The enzymes and peptides carried by the original cell of an individual or of a species are as important as the genetic pool carried by the cell in determining the characteristics of that individual or of that species.

It is the cell's enzymes which originate, carry on and terminate most of the activities of the cell. They are the cell's logic, language and grammar.

It is the cell's enzymes which activate and terminate the performance of the nuclear DNA, or nuclear genes. Without being stimulated, or irritated, by enzymes, genes would remain in their dormant state for ever.

It is the cell's enzymes which rule the activity of the cytoplasmic RNA, the second genetic code. In fact, RNA floating in the cytoplasm, and operated by the enzyme known as aminoacyl-transfer RNA synthetase, should be considered the first genetic code as, in evolutionary terms, it preceded DNA.

Due to their exceptional instability, therefore sensitivity and activity, cytoplasmic peptides play an important part in the growth of the cell. Any pressure or irritation of the cell increases the activity of the cell's peptides which stimulate the cell's growth.

The cell's answer to any pressure or irritation is its expansion. Growth is the main reaction of organic matter to irritation or pressure.

Becoming an integral part of a structure, the cell's components reduced their respective instabilities. Some components, like nuclear genes, even reached the dormant state of existence.

In becoming part of a whole, however, the cell's components also became a part of the instability of the complexity of the whole.

The main property of life is its reproduction. This was

originated and perpetuated by the cell's tendency to expand or grow under irritation or pressure.

At a certain stage of its growth, however, the cell became too big for its comfort. In order to lessen this discomfort of excessive growth, the cell released or rejected a part of itself, it divided into two cells.

We assume that the conditions and environment under which a cell divides must be ideal. In reality, however, the conditions and environment under which a cell divides should be irritating, as only the irritation of a cell could create its expansion or growth. A happy cell would never become two cells. A content caterpillar would never become a butterfly.

First Organisms

Monocellular organisms or bacteria appeared around 3.5 billion years ago.

The first bacteria consisted of procaryotic cells, or cells without nucleus, with their nucleic acids or genes floating in the cell's cytoplasm.

For the first 2.5 billion years, life on earth was dominated by procaryotic bacteria.

Around one billion years ago a more complex eucaryotic bacteria appeared, with their genes inside their nuclei, which were floating inside the cell's cytoplasm.

The eucaryotic cells presumably evolved from procaryotic cells, most probably from the more unstable and more vulnerable ones.

In search of lesser instabilities these more unstable procaryotic cells absorbed many enzymes, peptides, microbial compounds and a variety of RNA, so as to create more complex units. This complexity increased the cells' instabilities and vulnerabilities.

In these increased instabilities, the eucaryotic cells started forming symbioses with other more vulnerable bacteria such as mitochondria. Only a higher instability and a deeper vulnerability could have created a symbiotic relationship.

This became a turning point in the evolution of life.

With mitochondria's oxydative enzyme system, the eucaryotic cells were able to escape the dangerous environment dominated by the better organised procaryotic bacteria.

By carrying mitochondria, the eucaryotic cells could face the atmosphere with oxygen. By utilising oxygen, mitochondria became the power house of the eucaryotic cell.

In search of a lesser instability some eucaryotic cells started a symbiotic relationship with another highly unstable bacteria: chloroplasts, specialised in photosynthesis and in carbohydrates synthesis.

The eucaryotic cells' complexity increased their precariousness. In this increased precariousness, we might find the reason of the tendency of these eucaryotic cells to try to reduce their instability through assembling or aggregating into groups or colonies.

This tendency of the eucaryotic cells to try to reach a lesser precariousness through assembling, opened the way to the formation and the evolution of multicellular organisms.

Influenced by their gregarious cells, many of the multicellular organisms found their safety in numbers. Our present tendency to search for a lesser insecurity in togetherness and cuddling might easily be due to our eucaryotic cells' tendency to search for a lesser precariousness through physical contact.

A big, and in evolutionary terms sudden expansion of multicellular forms of life took place between 600 and 500 million years ago. This 'Cambrian explosion' was probably helped by the changes in climate. Another factor could also explain this explosion: an increase of oxygen in the atmosphere. Oxygen is irritating and irritation stimulates growth and expansion. In fact, respiration is not only important for the intake of oxygen but even more important in preventing too much of it, as taking in too much oxygen can be lethal for an organism.

That the formation of multicellular organisms was inspired and ruled by the instability of eucaryotic cells in search of a lesser instability can be seen in the fact that most multicellular organisms or structures tend to achieve the least possible assymetry of form.

There is an exception to every rule, there are still certain single eucaryotic celled organisms to-day.

This is probably due to the fact that their instability and their environment has not changed much since their origin.

Reproduction of life

An organism reaches its state of maturity, therefore its reproductive capacity, when it stops expanding or growing. We do not stop growing when we mature, we mature when we stop growing.

An organism stops growing when the potential of its cells becomes exhausted in a given environment. The growth of a living organism is an interplay between the biochemical potential of the original cell and the external forces operating in an environment.

If the environment was able to create life on earth, it is also able to influence its evolution.

Among the important forces influencing the growth of an organism are: degree of the sun's energy, humidity, atmospheric pressure, gravity, cosmic radiation and food availability.

There is a general belief that it is mainly genes which influence the development of the structural complexity of an organism. I think that it is the cell's use and manipulation of its genes that are the ruling factors in the development and the evolution of an individual's structural complexity. In spite of having more genetic material in their cells than humans, frogs and maize are structurally less complex.

On reaching its maturity, an organism starts its decline. Being irritating, therefore growth stimulating, exercises practiced by an organism in search of satisfying its elementary needs, can slow down the rhythm of the decline.

In certain special seasonal conditions, the first multi-cellular organisms in maturity developed an extra growth. Being a biological discomfort, this extra growth was ejected by the organism. From these ejected cells, in the correct environmental conditions, new organisms of the same species developed. Reproduction in nature is due to the ejection of extra growth.

The first multicellular organisms must have been androgynous, that is they must have been carrying characteristics of both sexes.

With the complexity brought by evolution, instability increased. In certain more unstable androgynous individuals, the characteristics of one sex, probably became more prominent. We should remember that any new step in evolution should be originated by a group of individuals which become more unstable than the rest of their species.

The male sex might have developed from androgynous individuals with an even deeper instability. That the male sex evolved from more unstable androgynous individuals can be deduced from the fact that the males of most species are bigger than females. This extra growth could only have been originated by a major biochemical instability in search of a lesser instability through expansion.

Carrying an increase in instability, any new phase in evolution tends to develop a kind of nostalgia towards the less unstable previous existence. Perhaps, this could explain the pairing of the sexes, male and female bonding, or humans' falling in love. Some humans reach a state of depression or despair when separated from their loved one.

In certain specific seasonal conditions, both males and females of the first bisexual species developed a marginal growth in their bodies, a growth of superfluous half cells, sex or germ cells, on maturing.

Creating an increase in biochemical discomfort, the body ejects these cells.

Guided by biochemical needs, nature has placed the glands where these extra sex cells are produced, either at the extreme end of the organism, or in the vicinity of the organs specialised for the evacuation of the body's waste, for easier ejection.

That the sex cells cause a biological irritation and discomfort can be seen by the distress in animals when on heat. In fact, it is this increase in instability, caused by the presence in the body of the extra sex cells, that provides the extra energy needed for sexual display, sexual fight or sexual intercourse.

That the sex cells are a nuisance can be seen by the fact that their presence stimulates the activity of the body's immune system.

That the presence in the body of the sex cells is a physiological discomfort can be seen by the obvious signs of relief in an animal after it has discharged them through sexual intercourse or otherwise.

In reality, the main purpose of sexual intercourse is not the fecondation and the reproduction of life, but the elimination of a biological discomfort, of an itch caused by the presence of irritating sex cells.

Fortunately for the reproduction of the bisexual species, these extra male and female sex cells, when ejected, and when meeting in their affinity and complementarity, unite, forming what we call a fertilised egg or a fertilised seed. In the right conditions, these fertilised eggs or seeds start producing a new organism.

Morphogenesis

How does an assembly of cells form an organism? What inspires a cell to specialise and form a different tissue, or the different organ of an organism?

The easy answer of many people is genes. This, however, does not answer a more serious question: what is it that triggers off the activity of a gene, and what is it that co-ordinates this activity.

In my view, the cell divides in order to aleviate its instability, it migrates driven by the same tendency, it settles following the same tendency, and it specialises in its activity in accordance with the same tendency. An organism is the result of a co-operative organisation of the cellular tendencies to reach their minimal instabilities.

Even some bacteria, these independent unicellular organisms, tend to reduce their individual instabilities by forming colonies, often even by forming communities, with their cellular interactions, the specialisations of some bacteria and the division of labour among them.

In an assembly of cells, each new cell or group of cells creates new conditions to which the rest of the cells have to adapt their constant tendency towards lesser discomfort. Each new group of cells is influenced by the previous cells and at the same time influences the state of existence and the metabolism of the previous cells of the organism.

Morphogenesis is a chain of successful organisms starting from the first division of the original cell to the final form. Each new group of cells created by the previous organism creates a new organism which, following its needs, will produce a new group of cells. A creation is influenced by its creator, but at the same time it influences its creator.

The idea of number might have been inspired in the brain by the eucaryotic cells' tendency to become a number and with the number to acquire a lesser instability in a multicellular organism.

By belonging to a group, each individual number acquires a co-operative meaning on the expenses of its individuality.

We are attracted by numbers, even if they show an increase in world population, or an increase in the population of our country or our town. So much for individuality.

Genes

Many people explain all things concerning the living world with genes. One has the impression that genes are a kind of omnipresent and omnipotent divinity. If a gene is not sufficient to explain something, the 'super gene' or 'master gene' intervene.

Believers of the omnipotence and omnipresence of genes call their belief 'genetic determinism'.

Each historic era has its favourite myth. The myth of the omnipotence of genes is very much in tune with the Western mentality influenced by the Judeo-Christian belief in a one and only omnipotent god.

As I said, people who insist that genes dictate everything do not explain, however, what it is that activates these genes. There is no scientific evidence that genes can start their own activity, their own self-actualisation. A cell is a co-operative organisation, and in a co-operation there is no room for determinisms.

I have explained that the drive inherent in organic matter forced genes into tightly compact chromosomes. Inside these chromosomes genes reach their minimal biochemical discomfort, a nesting or quiescent state of existence. Any separation of the chromosomes during the cell's division, or any revival of a gene situated on a chromosome would mean an increase in their instabilities which no organic molecule can do with its own initiative. An instability is always imposed by another major instability, a discomfort by another more irritating discomfort.

In order to become active a gene has to be activated.

What activates a gene?

The answer is the cell as a whole, as a co-operative organisation in which the most sensitive and the most unstable enzymes play an important part. It is, in fact, mainly enzymes which activate genes and which keep them active. As soon as an enzyme operating on a gene ceases its activity, the gene returns to its dormant state. It is also the enzyme that choses which gene, from maternal or paternal chromosomes, is better for the cell as a whole.

The genetic pool could be compared to a library where each reader choses his book following his needs of that moment. The more urgent the need of a reader, the more avidly he will search for the right book.

Geneticists stress that we inherit the genes of the species. But, we also inherit the cytoplasm of the species, we inherit the cell's membrane, with its receptors, of the species, we inherit mitochondria of the species, we inherit enzymes and the cell's organisation of the species.

With cytoplasm we also inherit the RNA of the species which plays an important role directly or indirectly in the synthesis of proteins.

For geneticists, the continuity of a species is due to the continuity of its genes. One can also add that the continuity of a species is due to the continuity of the cytoplasmic potential of that species. One could also add that the continuity of a species is also due to the continuity of the environmental conditions in which a species lives. A crocodile might have had many genetic mutations over the past two hundred million years, but crocodiles are still roughly the same.

Somehow, one has the impression that there is a kind of conspiracy among scientists, most of whom are men, to not mention all these inheritances and continuities as they are only passed through the female line. In the name of only half the genes which man provides to the genetic pool, he has invented genetic determinism. Aristotle who dominated and still dominates the western way of philosophising insisted that women contributed nothing to the reproduction of our species.

What geneticists also seldom mention is the fact that the first divisions of the cells at the beginning of the development of a new life are done under the influence of the cytoplasmic organisation of the egg, without any participation of the nucleic genes.

Perhaps, after all, taking into consideration the cytoplasmic organisation in the development of the organism, one can explain such a variety of species. We have, for instance, approx. 99% of genes in common with the chimpanzees. What makes us different is not so much that one per cent difference in the genes, but the difference in the cells organisations and their different manipulation of the genes that we do have in common.

In spite of having genetic pools in common, domestic animals are different in form and behaviour to their cousins in the wild.

There is evidence that the cells produced during the first steps of embryogenesis contain a variety of mediators, such as acetylcholine, dopamine, serotonine, adrenaline and noradrenaline. These mediators play an important role in the embryo's growth, the cells differentiation, their migration and their spacial orientation.

As these mediators are produced by the nervous system, a system as yet undeveloped in the embryo, we could conclude that they must have been provided by the mother through her egg's cytoplasm.

Geneticists insist that the evolution of the variety of species, plus the variety of individuals within each species, is mainly due to genetic mutations.

One could equally claim that it is also ruled by mutations in the species' cellular organisation, or mutations in the species' mitochondria. After all, mitochondria have their own genes and they synthetise their own proteins and enzymes independently. For instance, mitochondrial genes could explain these differences better than nucleic genes, particularly the differences among individuals of the same species, because the mutation rate of the former is about ten times higher than that of the latter. Individual energetic differences, so important in the intraspecific selection, are closely related to mitochondria, these power stations of the cell.

Geneticists also never admit that it is not the genes, but the cell as a whole, which manipulates the activity of its membrane's receptors, an activity of major importance as these receptors are in direct contact with the cell's environment.

We should never forget that life was created by the environmental conditions on our planet, and that life continues to be influenced by them. A small difference in the temperature of the incubation of many reptiles can determine their sex, completely ignoring their genes. In a colony of ants, where every individual has the same genes, it is environmental conditions which make some into queens, some into soldiers and some into workers.

It is the cell's organisation, stimulated by the external conditions and the cellular inherent drive towards a lesser biochemical instability, which operate cycles of DNA synthesis and the chromatine condensation in the division of cells.

If a mother, particularly during the first 12 weeks of pregnancy, even occasionally, takes cocaine, her child can easily be born deformed, without showing any mutation in his original genes inherited by his mother and his father. Deformities in the embryo were probably caused by the abnormal manipulation of genes by the embryo's cells, the abnormal activity of the embryo's cells having been produced by the cocaine, used by the mother. (Being soluble in fat, cocaine can easily cross the placenta of the mother's womb.)

The genetic pool can be enriched or mutated by the reverse transcription of viral or cytoplasmic RNA into the nucleic DNA, and this is performed by the cell's cytoplasm and by one of its specific enzymes, following their needs.

It is important to stress that nucleic genetic information has to be read and translated, and this is done by the cell's cytoplasm, mainly by its messenger RNA and its transfer RNA. After all, genes are letters which are picked up by enzymes and transformed by the cell's organisation into words, sentences, a meaningful text. Each cell has its own individual reading, its own writing, its own logic and style. These are related to the cell's degree of instability. The same cell is able to read and translate the same gene differently in different conditions, in different instabilities.

The collective memory of a species, and particularly the recognition and fear of natural enemies, must be passed to the new generation through the maternal eggs' cytoplasm and its enzymes and peptides.

Memorisation needs information. In order to become information or communication, an event must be perceived. Perception presupposes perceptivity and perceptivity is conditioned by alertness and vulnerability. Alertness and vulnerability are related to the state of instability.

Higher flexibility, a sign of higher instability of proteins, particularly of the enzymes and peptides, gives these proteins a major role in memorisation and learning. The energy for memorisation and learning can only be provided by instability.

Some genetic dogmatists insist that the whole life and its evolution only serve one purpose: that of the survival and propagation of the 'selfish gene'.

As a co-operative unit, the cell would never have been created with such a so-called selfish gene, in my view. What is more, if genes are selfish, therefore competitive, after four billion years of their competitive struggle some of them would be bigger than the Empire State Building by now.

One might also ask how a selfish gene could have exercised its selfishness when its selfish activity cannot take place without the intervention and help of enzymes of the co-operative cell.

In a co-operation there is no individual independence and without independence there can be no selfishness. Genes cannot be independent as they cannot survive without the cell.

If our brain cells were not co-operative by nature, we would not be able to create the idea of the division of labour and co-operation in economy.

Genetic determinism states that the cell can not alter its genetic constitution in the face of environmental changes.

The cell might not change the genetic constitution, but, with its enzymes, it can manipulate genes of the genetic pool following its needs ruled by the environmental conditions.

Behind the activity of a gene there is an enzyme, behind the activity of an enzyme there is the cell, with its organisation, influenced by the environmental conditions. This should be taken into consideration mainly because genetic mutations alone cannot explain such a variety of forms of life.

The dominance of genes is often called 'Central Dogma'. This idea of dogma was launched by Francis Crick, one of the discoverers of the DNA construction.

Judging by the book 'Origins' by Robert Shapiro, Crick did not know the real meaning of the word 'dogma'. 'I thought,' he said, 'it meant a hypothesis, some arbitrary thing which was laid down for no particular reason. Otherwise it would have been called the Central Hypothesis, and then nobody would have made all this fuss.'

Genetic determinism seems to have brought positive damage in the cure, and above all in the prevention, of cancer. Enormous resources have been spent in search of the gene causing the lethal disease. Many scientists are convinced they have found the cancer gene. They call it 'oncogene'.

Even if this oncogene existed, it must have been in our genetic pool for some time in a dormant state of existence. Perhaps, the real cause of cancer is not this quiescent oncogene, but the conditions which have forced the cell and its enzymes to revive and activate it from its dormant state.

With a wider approach, scientists might have discovered that the cell under tension, which increases its biochemical instability, tends to find a lesser instability through growth or expansion. They might have also discovered that, when irritated by external forces or by the mind's anxiety, an organism starts growing in its most unstable spot. An organism under stress develops a cancer of its most unstable cells. That is why the same kind of anxiety or stress can cause different cancers in different people.

The USA is investing around two billion dollars, and certain other countries are investing large amounts of resources, into providing geneticists with a new toy. With great euphoria, they are now preparing 'the handbook of man', a mapping project of all human genes.

'The handbook of man' will contain only letters. It will not, however, contain the explanation of what makes words from these letters, or what it is that makes sentences and text out of these words, and why.

Despite enormous research, there has been little progress in curing so-called genetic diseases. A less dogmatic approach to inherited deficiencies would have probably brought better results. In the obsession of finding the genes responsible for genetic diseases, and replacing them, two important facts are omitted to be considered.

First of all one should ask if the gene considered responsible for hereditary disease is actually unhealthy, or whether the gene was manipulated by its cell and the cell's enzymes in an abnormal way. One should then ask whether the cell and its enzymes would not also manipulate implanted or transplanted genes in the same way.

Gene obsession has distorted scientific research to such a point that some scientists are seriously trying to find 'genes for longevity'. For centuries, Medieval alchemists prospered by selling their 'elixir of eternal youth'.

Lately, there is talk about the 'obesity gene', supposed to be responsible for our over-weight.
We all know that in certain circumstances we put on weight, and in others we lose it. This happens without any change or mutation in our genes. We all also know that the mind and its anxieties can be a major factor in people's obesity, as well as in anorexia nervosa, or other psychosomatic disorders or diseases.

The most important evidence that my theory of dormant genes is valid can be seen in the synthesis of the stress or shock proteins. An increase in the strength of stressful environmental factors such as heat, pollution, lack of oxygen, exposure to heavy metals or poisonous chemicals and physical trauma, can trigger off the activity of the suitable gene so that it helps the synthesis of an appropriate stress protein which would enable the cell or the organism to resist the external stress more successfully. Without the stressful environmental factors, the genes helping the synthesis of the stress proteins would remain dormant for ever.

Why is there this passion for gene dominance?
It is very much in tune with the adolescent mentality,

of lonely and isolated individuals, to solve everything through a 'one and only' individual cause. (Later I will explain that we are dominated by the adolescent mentality).

It is this mentality which invented monotheism. In the Middle Ages everything was explained by the supreme god. The scientific XIX Century, and the first half of this Century, tried to explain everything with mythic instincts. Nowadays everything is seen in a key of genes.

Many are convinced that there are genes for aggression, violence and crime. Before genes were invented, aggression, violence and crime were attributed to the mystic power of instincts. Some scientists and politicians insisted, and some still insist, that wars are a necessity, that they are good and healthy for the discharge of instinctive aggressiveness. This is believed in spite of the fact that most violence and crime is premeditated, often even efficiently and rationally planned. But, the inability to grasp facts is in the nature of stubborn believers.

The adolescent mentality also invented the idea of a scapegoat, which is blamed for everything. After all, the adolescent mentality is a pretentious and capricious mentality.

The major evidence that the 'omnipotence' of the 'selfish gene' is an adolescent mentality's myth is the fact that it is the cell as a whole which provides the conditions and energy needed by the DNA to make copies of itself during the cellular reproduction.

Evolution

We are accustomed to considering evolution as a progress, a development from lower to higher forms of life. These higher forms of life would have been mainly created by genetic mutations, coupled with natural selection. Having a better chance of survival and reproduction, the fittest would transmit their fitness to their descendents. In the Darwinian sense, evolution works upwards.

This idea was probably inspired by the fact that evolution brings more and more complex forms of life, and complexity tends to impress us.

Being a product of instability, any evolution of complexity only increases instability. With the human mind, this latest achievement in evolution, instability often reaches panicky or suicidal precariousness.

In fact, we seem to have achieved decline rather than evolution, taking into consideration that complexity increases instability which tries to lessen itself through expansion or growth, thus increasing complexity and vulnerability. The human brain would never have been able to invent the idea of the 'good old days' if evolution was bringing more stability.

Complexity increases instability and vulnerability because it increases needs and demands.

When the needs of complexity become superior to its benefices, the decline starts. Every form of life starts decaying when its expansion has created the needs and demands beyond its ability to cope with them. Dinosaurs could be an example of how expansion reached its over-expansion, bringing the fall.

It is in the nature of expansion to result in over-expansion. It is in the nature of over-expansion to break into a decline, and it is in the nature of a decline to eventually end. Life dies of its natural disease: over-expansion.

In a certain sense, we realise the increase in instability and vulnerability with evolution by noticing an increase in the sensitivity to pain with higher forms of life. This sensitivity to pain often reaches hysterical proportions with man.

Creating an increase in complexity and precariousness, evolution also increases fears. With human consciousness, evolution brought fear of ageing and fear of death. With the evolution of the mind, anxiety and stress appeared, and with the evolution of the inflated ego, mental suffering developed. With imagination fear of ghosts appeared.

Being more complex, higher forms of life are more susceptible to a greater variety of diseases. With the evolution of the mind, we became susceptible to all kinds of psychosomatic diseases, mental disorders and suicide. The continuous increase in alcohol consumption and drug addiction is clear evidence of the continuous increase in instability, fears and anxieties.

It is an established belief that life and its evolution run counter to the Second Law of Thermodynamics, which involves the concept of entropy.

But, is the order of life really in contravention with this law?

The order of life seems to be in harmony with the Second Law of Thermodynamics if we take into consideration that, through its growth and expansion, life evolves towards its decline. What is more, life's expansion and growth reduce the conditions for life on this planet. Over the last hundred million years there were more species which disappeared than those which appeared. In the last hundred years the list of the endangered species is progressively getting longer. Life itself seems to be more and more in danger.

As far as the theory of the survival of the fittest is concerned, one could say that it sounds more accurate than it really is.

We consider it logical that the fittest survives better. We do not, however, give a definition of the fittest. We simply consider that those who survive best must be the fittest.

Presumably the fittest are those who are successful in life. In order to be successful, one needs more energy, more aggressiveness, more competitiveness, more ruthlessness and more callousness. This can only be provided by an above-average instability and vulnerability. In fact, evolution seems to produce ever increasing complexities which implies ever increasing instability and vulnerability.

In humans, this latest achievement of evolution, where an individual ego plays an important role in sexual competition and reproduction, we see those with more fragile egos, therefore more in need of personal success, being more successful in seducing, or assaulting, and reproducing, than the people with less unstable egos, than wise and intelligent people.

What is more, this mind's survival and the survival of its inflated ego can seriously endanger life in general.

The theory of the survival of the fittest always reminds me of the story of an Italian doctor. In a hospital in Genoa, two terminal cancer cases, Mario and Gino, shared a room. Mario who was near the window used to spend hours entertaining Gino, in the far corner of the room, by depicting life and the goings on in the street below. One night Mario was in agony. Gesticulating, he begged Gino to call the nurse. Gino decided not to call the nurse because he wanted to take his bed and spend the rest of his days watching the life outside.

When Gino settled into Mario's bed, he looked out of the window. There was no street outside, and nothing going on.

Evolution of humans

My theory that a new species mainly evolves from the more unstable group of individuals of the species, is best illustrated in the evolution of the human species.

It is estimated that the creation of earth took place about 4,500 million years ago. Approximately 4,000 million years ago the sea was formed. Soon after the first life appeared in the water in the form of single-celled algae and bacteria. Around 1,000 million years ago oxygen-breathing multicellular organisms started evolving. The development of various forms of fish took place 600–400 million years ago. 430 million years ago land plants began to grow. Between 400 and 300 million years ago amphibians, reptiles and insects started evolving. Approximately 230 million years ago the dinosaurs appeared, followed by mammals and birds.

Any increase in the instability of individuals belonging to a species creates the tendency to search for a lesser instability by escaping from the pressure of the rest of the species. From the escape of the eucaryotic cell from the dominating procaryotic bacteria, the escape is the important factor in the evolution of the new species. The ancestors of reptiles must have escaped from their better equipped cousins of the sea, the ancestors of mammals from reptiles, the ancestors of primates from mammals, and the ancestors of humans from primates. It is in the nature of an escape to be forced on the escapee.

The new and irritating conditions of escape stimulate the development of complexities, the characteristic of any new step in evolution.

Around 70 million years ago, the ancestors of our ancestors, small, ratlike insectivores, left their perilous life on the ground for a safer one up in the trees. In these small, tree-shrew type of mammals, who chose an arboreal environment for reason of safety, we find the origins of the primates. The first page of the history of mankind opens in the woodlands of East Africa.

Carlton S. Coon reflects the present scientific attitude concerning the evolution of humans when in his book 'The History of Man' he reduced the evolution of our species to the following three sentences: 'From some kind of a Miocene ape probably living in Africa, both living apes and men are descended. The apes' ancestors, after a trial period on the ground, swung back into the trees. Ours stayed below, rose onto their hind-legs, made tools, walked, talked and became hunters.'

In other words, humans and apes decided one day to come down from the trees, to leave an environment ideal from the point of view of food and safety. Then the apes, the less advanced animals, returned to the trees and lived happily ever after, while the more advanced humans walked out of their natural paradise into the hell of the savannah.

In the savannah, our human ancestors, with no natural specialisation, small and fragile, with a brain not more than a third of the size of a gorilla today (i.e. one seventh the capacity of that of modern man), had to live and compete with specialised and dangerous predators. We must remember that originally the ancestors of primates fled from the dangerous ground into the safety of the trees, a wise step which must have left a trace on their brains. No animal will ever willingly leave a safe environment for a dangerous one, especially when it has an inbuilt fear of the danger. This inborn fear of falling is occasionally experienced in our nightmares.

I think that the following explanation of the evolution of humans would be more plausible than the self-glorifying one we prefer.

In the Eocene epoch (58–36 million years ago) there was already a distinction between anthropoids and prosimians. The former were humanlike primates, the latter included the ancestors of lemurs, tarsiers, and tree-shrews.

In the Oligocene epoch (36–25 million years ego), human and apes' ancestors lived together in an abundance of food and safety.

In the Miocene epoch (26–13 million years ago) a major event occured in the evolution of mankind: a change of climate took place. The deterioration of atmospheric conditions transformed a great part of the woodlands into a savannah. During the long phase of this change, being more fragile, our ancestors were forced to abandon the woodlands and face the life of the savannah, to escape from the pressure of the better equipped apes.

Mankind is the product of neither fallen angels nor elevated apes. Mankind stems from fallen apes. The Bible is more accurate than science in its explanation of the origin of human life. Our ancestors, our Adams and Eves, were evicted from Paradise. The only difference is that they were not evited by Almighty God, but by fitter apes.

By the close of the Miocene era, our ancestors were living in the savannah, about to confront the Pliocene epoch, which lasted 13–1 million years ago. This was the most testing time in the history of mankind – an era of climatic deteriorations and droughts which transformed Africa into a graveyard for many species. This climatically aggressive situation must have left a deep scar on the human brain, a scar which must have influenced the mind in its creation of the first idea of hell. It says, in the Sumerian epic 'Inanna's Journey to Hell': 'Here is no water but only rock, rock and no water and the sandy road' . . .

In 'The Epic of Gilgamesh' the writer states that 'Hell is frightening because of its sandy dust' . . It is 'the river which has no water.'

In order to escape from the woodlands into the savannah, our ancestors must have been more undeveloped than the rest of the apes.

Even today, most scientists agree that we are in a phase of infancy or neoteny. 'The characteristic which is so vital for the peculiarity of true man, that of always remaining in a state of development, is quite certainly a gift we owe to the neotenous nature of mankind,' writes K. Lorenz.

To be in a 'state of development' one has to be in an undeveloped state. In fact, even today, an adult human being looks more like an infant chimpanzee than an adult chimpanzee. Our ancestors may have never developed canine teeth.

Life in the savannah produced two important changes in the evolution of our species: the enlargement of the brain and the upright posture or bipedalism.

The permanent frustration caused by the new environment of the savannah produced a constant pressure on our ancestors' brain cells, causing their growth, and the increase in the volume of the human brain. Irritation is one of the major causes of expansion and growth in nature.

By carrying frustration, each escape produced an increase in the volume of the brain. The reptilian brain is bigger than that of fishes, the mammalian bigger than that of reptiles, the primate's bigger than that of the rest of the mammals, and the human brain is bigger than that of primates.

Around one million years ago, the brain of our ancestors reached the size of 1.300 cubic centimetres.

In the same period our ancestors became bipedal creatures. Homo became erectus.

There are a variety of theories trying to explain the reason for human upright posture. Some writers believe that our bipedalism was the result of the need to free the hands in order to use weapons and tools better. Evidence, however, shows that man did not start using weapons and tools efficiently until long after he had been standing upright. Weapons and tools, such as they were at the beginning of man's bipedalism, were used with equal dexterity by apes.

Some writers explain that man became upright because from the new posture he could spot his prey more easily.

Would it not be more in tune with the natural logic that a highly vulnerable creature like man, with no offensive or defensive weapons, and lacking the speed of other animals, would have been much more worried about being seen by his predators than spotting his prey. After all, at the start of their bipedalism, humans were more food gatherers than hunters.

Some writers even explain that our ancestors assumed the upright posture in order to have frontal copulation which would be more in tune with the human dignity of their descendents.

What happened then?

The upright posture must have been forced on humans. It is not in the nature of an animal to assume a precarious and uncomfortable posture unless it is to avoid or escape from an even more uncomfortable one.

In order to understand the reason for the human upright posture, we must take into consideration that the upright posture coincided with the increase in volume, therefore weight, of the human brain.

The phases of gradual bipedalism followed the stages of the gradual increase in the size of the brain. And so it would seem that the human erect posture was due to the extra weight in the head. Erect posture was not a choice of man but was forced on him. It was forced on him by the extra weight – approximately 800 grams – of the new brain.

It may seem unbelievable that this small weight could

have produced such consequences. It would probably have been irrelevant had it been carried on four legs for a short time, but for a long time, coupled with the exhaustion of food gathering in the savannah, this small weight felt heavy.

Under the pressure of the increased weight of their brain, humans had to stand upright in order to reduce discomfort by balancing the head on the spinal cord.

We can deduce that the upright posture was forced on humans from the fact that it has brought illnesses, such as curvature of the spine, back pains, kidney troubles, and varicose veins.

The upright posture brought some changes in blood circulation. In the new body position, circulation of blood to the new brain became more difficult. This increased mental fatigue which might have influenced the efficiency of the senses and of perception.

Many scientists explain that we are a neotenous or infantile species. If we are a neotenous species, then we must have been even more so in the past. If we were a neotenous species in the past, it seems logical that we lived in a group, and were guided and ruled by our mothers. Most women acquire a certain maturity with pregnancy and motherhood, maturity implying the protection and care of infants, so necessary for a neotenous species.

There is, in fact, positive evidence that we entered history as a species dominated by mothers.

How then did this mothers' rule, which enabled the human species to survive for so many millions of years, get destroyed? What was responsible for changing the inoffensive groups of food gatherers into hordes and gangs of violent and aggressive killers?

The answer can only be: the mind of the adolescent male.

Our species must have always had a long adolescence,

more pronounced in males than in females.

Adolescence is basically a state of increased instability. An increase in instability carries an increase in restlessness and agitation. Sooner or later, however, the group must have cooled down most of these restless adolescents, giving them their place and rank in the community.

The more unstable and more agitated individuals, however, who were unable to adapt to the established order of the group, were either alienated or opted out of the group.

These lonely and frightened adolescents, living on the edge of the communities, started forming gangs. These gangs created a radical change in the life of the human species, gradually replacing the community with gang mentality.

With their, what could be called 'adolescent revolutions', slowly but surely, they replaced the natural order based on the mother-infant relationship, with their own order, based on an artificial father-infant relationship.

These adolescent revolutions took place between twelve and two thousand years ago. Five thousand years ago, in the Vinca area of Central Serbia, and the Sesklo area in Northern Greece, evidence of the adolescent revolutions unearthed figurines of male nudes, proudly holding penises were already in prominence. In the same period the Mesopotamian myth tells that the first male divinity, Marduk, had to kill his mother in order to get power. By the Sixth Century B.C., Greece achieved male supremacy. Women became the main characters of Greek tragedies. With Judeo-Christianity, the total subordination of woman was institutionalised.

Where and how did these adolescents find the audacity to challenge the established order which had cared for our species for so long? Where and how did they find their aggressiveness and the temerity to use force against the natural laws and rules? Above all, where and how did they find their aggressiveness and the temerity to use force against the natural laws and rules? Above all, where and how did these adolescents find the extra energy to feed their audacity, their aggressiveness and their violence?

The adolescents found their audacity, their aggressiveness and the temerity to use it against the natural laws and rules in the agitation and restlessness caused by increased instability.

These alienated and lonely individuals also found the extra energy needed to feed their audacity, their aggressiveness and their violence, in this increased instability and fear.

The increased instability and fear increased the instability of our ancestors' sensory and perceptive systems creating doubt and uncertainty. This created a new brain's mental activity, an activity based on approximations, assumptions, hypotheses and speculation. This mental activity, based on the reduced efficiency of the sensory and perceptive systems, created by the increase in the instability, is what we call the mind.

In search of lesser discontent, the mind started escaping into wishful thinking, which produced hopeful beliefs. Hopeful beliefs could only have been developed with reduced sensory and perceptive efficiencies, caused by the increased instability. Only reduced or confused sensory and perceptive efficiencies of our brain could have allowed imagination, speculation and fantasies to take place.

In his fantasy, the adolescent replaced his inadequate self with a wishful idea of self, with an 'ought to be' self, with an idealised ego

When the adolescent invented his idealised ego, he became infatuated by it. It is in the nature of a creator to fall in love with his creation.

With self-love, the adolescent 'I' became the centre of the universe. That is probably why scientists have invented the so-called 'Anthropic Principle' which stresses that without man there would not be the universe, that it is man who brings the universe into existence. That is probably why humanity took so long to discover a Copernicus. In the English language, 'I' is still a capital letter.

An infatuated ego is an inflated ego. In nature inflation is usually caused by an increase in fears. Animals magnify their aspects when afraid.

With the mind's escape into its wishful thinking, and with the mind's created idealised ego, a new order in the universe started, an order which tries to find a lesser instability in trying to change the universe.

The order of the mind evolved from the order of organic matter. The new order carries an increase in the instability over the previous order. This increased instability brought a unique behaviour: a persistent tendency to force nature to fit super-nature, to change objective reality to suit subjective idealisations.

The order of the mind is a destructive order. One can only realise an idealisation at the expense of reality, and this can only increase precariousness and instability.

Anxiety

One could ask why, if humans so enjoy living in their imaginary world of the mind, they are not happier?

With adolescence, we start taking the world of the mind too seriously. Children and even mature men and women also develop certain fantasies, but they play with them.

Taking the world of the mind too seriously, created an abstract seriousness which I would like to call over-seriousness, as it is in the nature of abstractions to exaggerate: with exaggeration, abstractions hope to become reality. This makes over-seriousness not serious, therefore, a source of the ridiculous.

By taking the mind over-seriously, the human natural jovial, vivacious and flexible face and body disappear, and are replaced by over-seriousness, stiffness and tension. Many of the hard lines or distortions on a face are carved by a stubborn belief, by arrogant prejudice or by an aggressive concept of superiority.

How can the wishful thinking of the mind create tension? How can the mind's prejudices and beliefs create the necessary energy for their realisation?

By escaping from reality into the wishful world of the mind, we develop that brooding apprehension of the failure of our wishful expectations and hopes. We develop a dread that our pretensions, our longings and yearnings may not materialise. We develop the threat of reality. We develop anxiety.

In its complexity, the mind is unable to realise that its pretensions and hopes, its longing and yearning can only increase the instability.

Dante was mistaken when he stressed that hell was the place where there is no hope. In reality, anxiety caused by pretentious hopes is hell.

Awareness of the mind's created anxiety, like the awareness of a real fear, triggers off a state of alarm or emergency.

Like a real fear, the mind's created anxiety stimulates our hypothalamus. The hypothalamus, which controls our autonomic nervous system, triggers off the activity of the sympathetic system, and through the pituitary gland, activates the secretion of the adrenaline and noradrenaline.

Through the pituitary gland, our hypothalamus can also activate the thyroid gland which increases the rate of oxidative processes and metabolism, improving the body's state of energy.

Released by the activated sympathetic system, the neurotransmitters accelerate the heartbeat and increase the blood pressure.

Adrenaline increases the oxygen consumption at the tissue level, stimulates the heart, increasing cardiac output, and raises the level of energy providing glucose in the blood, thereby improving the tonus of the voluntary muscles, creating readiness for action.

Noradrenaline re-inforces the blood pressure by narrowing the peripheral blood vessels and small arteries. It also widens the arterioles of the voluntary muscles, essential for a quick and decisive reaction.

The neurotransmitters of the sympathetic nervous system and the hormones of the adrenal and thyroid glands, therefore, mobilise a chain of the body's cells, imposing extra activity on them. Nature provides this mechanism to create extra energy and readiness to enable an individual to solve the problem of a sudden temporary alarm or emergency, through the philogenetically programmed drives of fight or flight.

With its persistent wishful ideas and its persevering hopeful prejudices and beliefs, our mind, however, creates a lasting apprehension, a protracted dread of defeat, a constant anxiety. Self-love, self-infatuation, wishful expectations and hopeful beliefs are permanently under threat in the mind of the beholder. The world of beliefs is constantly shadowed by that important source of anxiety: imaginary demons or dark forces.

The lasting apprehensions of our mind's world and the protracted dread of the defeat of our self-created self can produce a more or less permanent state of alarm or anxiety, which results in a more or less permanent tension. Not being discharged in fight or flight, this tension becomes a biological discomfort, an inner irritation. This tension or arousal is commonly known as nervous energy.

A real fear and the mind's created anxiety seldom coexist. By eliminating the ego, a real fear also eliminates the mind's anxiety. In fact, anxiety related mental disorders can be placated with realistic problems or positive fears. Many anxiety-caused mental disorders disappear during wars or catastrophes.

On the other hand, high anxiety can reduce the efficiency of the senses and perception to the point of inability to sense or perceive real danger.

With the appearance of the mind and its wishful beliefs, inner tension also increased because the mind's world, dominated by the ego, started inhibiting the limbic brain, controlling or repressing its emotions and their discharge, thus increasing nervous energy. Before the appearance of the mind, human behaviour was mainly the result of a spontaneous intuitive reaction, intuition being the brain's perception of its cells' states of existence and tendency, caused by a sensation.

With the mind's world of beliefs prayer appeared. The adolescent minded started praying to supernatural forces to help realise their pretensions. The energy needed for prayer was provided by the anxiety that our hopes and expectations might not be fulfilled. With the mind's wishful thinking, belief in miracles became logical.

Anxiety is the price we pay for living in the world of imagination and fantasies, by living dangerously in the uncertain world of the mind created by wishful thinking.

The wider the discrepancy between our pretensions and our ability to reach them, the bigger our anxiety. This anxiety can be increased by either increasing our pretensions, or by decreasing our abilities. We can increase our pretentiousness by acquiring new political or economic rights, by a higher standard of living, by trying to acquire cultural, technological or scientific achievements, or by magnifying our self-infatuation and self-importance.

Our ability and potential diminishes with tiredness, invalidness, political or economic restrictions, a new environment, being a minority in a community, and by losing a loved one.

Causing a biological discomfort and inner irritation, the anxiety's created nervous energy craves discharge.

It is in this nervous energy that the lonely adolescents found their audacity, aggressiveness and strength to challenge the universe with its own natural orders.

It is this nervous energy which helped the adolescent minded to impose themselves on the rest of humanity.

In order to understand the nature of anxiety's generated nervous energy better, I would like to briefly mention the nature of the energies of the other two major groups of humans.

We have juvenile or child-like humanity with its energy generated by natural exuberance and playfulness, and we have the energy of maturity, generated by maturity's fecundity and fruitfulness. Maturity implies maternity. In fact, in maturity even the male becomes maternal and caring.

While juvenile energy and the energy of maturity are limited by the biological potentials of their carriers, nervous energy can go beyond this potential, often damaging its carrier biologically, because the source of this energy, which is the mind's anxiety, can be limitless.

Nervous energy, juvenile energy and the energy of maturity could be illustrated through a musician playing his instrument.

Usually living in a juvenile state of existence, within a community dominated by mothers, a gypsy musician will play with his instrument as if it was his toy. The adolescent minded person will perform on his instrument. A musician in maturity will communicate with his instrument, often with the virtuosity of magnanimity. When Jewish Kibbutzim started it was organised and run by the energies of juvenile and mature mentalities. It is changing radically since the increasing appearance of the adolescent mentality among its members.

The adolescent mentality's audacity became a uniqueness in nature. It was an irrational phenomenon as it was not in natural logic to provoke the established rules of nature. The adolescent mentality's culture glorified and still glorifies audacity. Some even consider audacity a virtue, a virtue favoured by fortune.

In order to justify audacity and the aggression, which usually accompanies it, the adolescent mentality's culture and science explain that they are our instincts, our genetic inheritance, part of our nature.

In my view, audacity and aggression are products of the adolescent mentality. After all, most audacities and aggressions are premeditated by a pretentious or self-righteous ego.

If nature had given audacity and aggression to the human species as instincts or innate drives, then nature must have been a practical joker giving us instincts without providing natural or innate weapons to exercise them.

We use a variety of stimulants which help to increase our nervous energy, our audacity and our aggressiveness.

Most of these stimulants are irritants which generate discomfort or unease and these create anxiety which produce nervous energy, restlessness, agitation, audacity and aggression.

The new order of the mind brought the following novelties which are typical of humanity dominated by the adolescent mentality: alcoholism, drugs, corruption, perversion, rape, sadism, torture, envy, jealousy, vindictiveness, fanaticism, obsessions, obstinancy, malevolence, self-deceptions, ideological and religious persecutions and wars.
Strong anxieties or stress also brought cardiovascular problems, psychosomatic diseases, cancers, immunodeficiency, mental disorders, sexual deviations, obesity, anorexia nervosa and suicide.

The wide range of emotional states, generated by the vast range of anxieties, contributed to the development and the richness of that specific uniqueness in nature: language. Through the human voice, the mind's world hopes to become reality. The urge of the image is to become 'the word'.
The energy needed by speech is mainly provided for by anxiety created nervous energy. In fact, speech is often used as a means of discharging this nervous energy. One has only to attend a cocktail party to realise this.
That human language is related to anxieties can be deduced from the fact that people living in areas with lesser anxieties have poorer vocabularies.
When a real problem or a positive fear eliminates the mind's world with its anxieties, our language is reduced to gesticulations.
By reducing the mind's world and its anxieties, physical fatigue can also reduce the use of a language.
Each individual has his own personal language. This language reflects that of the individual's mind. This

mind's language is influenced by the brain's activity in search of a lesser instability. The rhythm of this activity is mainly ruled by the most unstable component of the brain's cells, the most unstable component of the brain's cells varying from individual to individual.

Many national languages reflect national anxieties. Regional dialects can reflect regional anxieties. Jargons reflect the anxieties of a specific gang or community even more.

Having abstract values, therefore similar anxieties in common, creates the essential conditions for a language in common.

Participating in the culture and values, therefore in the anxieties of a foreign nation, greatly facilitates the learning of that nation's language. A fervent believer in the superiority of his own national values and culture rarely learns a foreign language fluently. A fervent believer in the superiority of his national values and culture, however, can become rich in his own language, as strong beliefs are rich in anxieties.

Following the 'ought to be' wishful ideas, the new humanity started assuming attitudes.

Animals' behaviour is in accordance with their biological age and stage. With humans, behaviour is mainly in accordance with mental attitudes. Mental attitudes became determining factors of human style of life and behaviour. Mental attitudes or mentalities became determinant factors in human behaviour because of their capacity to influence the brain's glandular activity, its secretion of hormones and neurotransmitters. This can best be seen in human sexual behaviour and sexual deviations in which the mind plays an essential role.

With the mind's wishful thinking, maturity no longer comes naturally with adulthood. Even the elderly can remain in an adolescent frame of mind until they die.

On the other hand, some people keep their juvenile

mentality all their lives, while others, mainly mothers, live theirs with a mature mentality.

Many people, and inside a short period of time, can switch from one mentality to another. A person with a juvenile mentality, in a moment of self-infatuation, can acquire an adolescent mentality, and in a moment of being needed, a caring, a mature mentality. At the time of the gratification of his ego, a person with an adolescent mentality can become benevolent and mature. When suitably shaken or degraded in his wishful beliefs, someone with an adolescent mentality can acquire either a juvenile or a mature mentality. In fact, as most crimes are committed by people with adolescent mentalities, the punishment is supposed to shake their self-righteous egos in order to bring them either to the flexible juvenile mentality or to the tolerance and understanding of the mature mentality.

Mentality can be influenced by many things: inner vulnerability, culture, environment, political or economic circumstances, and above all, by conditions of health. An acquired title or diploma can also change a mentality into another. An aggressive trade unionist in Britain can acquire a mature mentality when he becomes a member of the House of Lords.

In the last fifty years we have a fast rising mentality of old age pensioners. Some of them acquire a kind of 'après moi le déluge' mentality.

Political terror can push many towards a paranoic mentality.

Inside any mentality, and above all inside the adolescent mentality, lie a vast range of degrees of that mentality.

With such a variety of mentalities to influence human behaviour, it seems rather ridiculous to talk, like many scientists do, about human nature. With such a variety of mentalities, any economic or political theory, based on the 'eternal and immutable laws of human nature' is pointless.

Each mentality, and each degree of the same mentality, have their own way of reasoning. Each mentality, and each degree of the same mentality, have their own ideas of freedom, and their own ways of pursuing it. Each mentality, and each degree of the same mentality, have their own concepts of happiness and contentment, and their own ways of pursuing them. The same goes for: tolerance, justice, wisdom, peace, beauty, duty, family, immortality and death, pleasure and pain, virtue and vice, time and a sense of organisation.

Dominated by the adolescent mentality, our culture and science insist, for instance, that selfishness and aggression are in human nature. They are, in fact, in the nature of the adolescent mentaity. We seldom, however, see selfishness and aggression in the playfulness of the juvenile mentality or in the serenity and magnanimity of the mature mentality.

Conflicts within the human species are mainly caused by the misunderstandings or non-understandings among different mentalities, or among different degrees of the same mentality.

The closest understanding occurs among individuals with the juvenile mentaity, and among individuals with the mature mentality, particularly among mature women. There is also a great deal of understanding between individuals with the juvenile mentality and those with the mature mentality. Individuals with the adolescent mentaity communicate mainly with their own personal egos, listening mainly to their mind's wishfulness.

With the appearance of mentalities, dealing with human evolution became rather confusing. Perhaps we should deal with the evolution of human mentalities instead.

Humanity became seduced by the adolescent mentality mainly because it gives the impression of providing a more intensive and more interesting life. We pay for this intensive and interesting life with anxiety.

Perhaps, the Chinese malediction: 'May you have an interesting life,' really means: 'May you have an agitated life'.

Anxiety and the span of life

With the new order of the mind and its nervous energy, produced by anxieties, humanity became the most restless and the most agitated species on the planet. A great deal of human activities became related to the discharge of their nervous energies. As a result of this, humanity started producing the unnecessary, the superfluous.

That a great deal of human activities are more stimulated by restlessness and agitation than by rational reasoning is best seen in the arts, science and technology, which have advanced way beyond our needs, and in certain fields dangerously so.

We are proud of our progress, above all when this progress is unnecessary or superfluous. Our mind invokes pride whenever it has to placate its suspicion about its rationality.

Could it not be that anxiety caused agitations have produced another unnecessary phenomenon: life after the end of its reproductive capacities?

In my view, it is nervous energy, restlessness and agitation, created by anxiety, which has contributed a great deal to the longer span of life, particularly in the West. In fact, our span of life started lengthening in the West with the increase in anxieties created by the Western mind and its values, particularly over the last two centuries. Until the French Revolution of 1789, which opened an era of increasing uncertainties and anxieties, the average span of life had been about 35–40 years for centuries. In Western Europe and North America to-day life expectancy is around 72–75 years.

To the increase of anxiety in the last two centuries, a great deal of uncertainty and loneliness, brought on by urbanisation and industrialisation, contributed.

How can anxieties contribute to prolonging life?

The answer to this question is simple. Anxiety, particularly in moderation, prolongs life by stimulating life.

Nervous energy and agitation, brought on by anxieties, keep the body and the brain busy and active, often under constant exercises, which slows down decay or ageing. An organism starts decaying or ageing when its expansion or growth end, which is at around twenty years of age in our species.

Most people claim that the improved standard of living and advanced medicine have mainly contributed to the longer span of life of inhabitants of the Western World.

But, could it not also be that anxieties with their nervous energy and agitation, that created this better standard of living and this better medicine, were also contributing to the longer span of life in the West, by keeping people mentally and physically active, even if these activities were often unnecessary?

It is a known fact that many creative people live long. Constant creativity is the result of constant anxieties and the energies they generate.

Stopping their professional life with its anxieties, retired people often start ageing rapidly.

The same anxieties which slow down the ageing process, preventing death from old age, have, however, brought their own forms of death. These mainly consist of the breaking down of an over-active organism through heart collapse, or through an uncontrolled growth of some cells under excessive pressure, or through opportunistic infections, infections exploiting the body's reduced immunoefficiency.

We complain about the increase in anxiety-related heart disease, cancer, or opportunistic infections, but in most cases it is the same anxieties which break down long life that also created that long life.

Stress, which is produced by an extreme range of anxieties, can anticipate or accelerate the breaking down of an organism. Stress takes place any time the mind's pretentions or ambitions significantly exceed an individual's mental and physical capabilities to cope with them, creating damaging irritation or frustration.

While, in their moderate range, anxieties can be constructive and creative, stress is always consuming, destructive or damaging. Stress' consequences are usually beyond repair.

There is evidence that excessive radiation, which is a form of stress and irritation, can cause cancer. But, irritating animals with moderate radiation has shown that it prolongs their lives.

Anxieties also extend life by reducing sleeping hours. Without some anxieties many people would spend most of their time lying languidly in bed. How many of us would get up before midday without some anxieties?

In nature, the older an animal, the longer it sleeps. In the human species, however, with its new order of the mind and with the mind's anxieties, the older a person, the less he sleeps.

But, are we really prolonging life, or are we placed in an illusion by the specific characteristic of our species: self-deception?

We have achieved a longer span of life, but we have less time to live life, less time to give time, less time to play with time.

We have no time to love time, to share time. We have no time to mature, we have no time to reason reasonably; we reason under the pressure of urgency.

We spend all our time in rushing, rushing for more time, without realising that rushing kills time, rushing us out of time, out of living.

We may exist longer, but we live less, devoid of time.

Anxiety and growth

Attracting blood with its food and oxygen, an irritation can enlarge an organism or a part of it. The tendency of cells under pressure is to try to find a lesser discomfort through growth. The whole process of healing and self-repair is based on this tendency. By increasing the instability and discomfort of the cells, a wound or a cut in a body, increases the cells tendency to find a lesser instability or a lesser discomfort through expansion or growth. We scratch the dormant parts of our body in order to put pressure on their cells, and revive them.

If an irritation can increase growth, then, being an irritation, anxiety should be able to do the same, it should be able to contribute to the development of height and the weight of an organism.

Our species has the widest range of differences in height and weight than any other species.

Most scientists explain that these differences are due to the individual differences in genes, genes for height and genes for weight. On that basis, surely, our cousins, the chimpanzees must also have differences in their individual genes for height and weight, but there is little difference in their individual sizes.

I think that such important individual differences in height and weight in our species could be better explained stressing that these differences are not due so much to genetic differences among individuals, but more to the differences of an individual's activation and use of these genes.

If the cells of a developing organism are more under pressure they will keep the growth gene of that organism more active, creating a taller individual.

If the cells of a developing organism are less irritated, the organism will tend to be less tall and less heavy.

Experiments have proved that under certain irritation from mild doses of radiation, animals show an increase in their rate of growth and development.

In my view, the wide range of individual height and weight in humans is mainly due to anxieties and their powers of irritation.

There is a direct and permanent relationship between the mind with its anxieties and the hypothalamus. This important gland of our brain is in direct and permanent contact with the pituitary gland where the secretion of growth hormones takes place. By stimulating the activity of the hypothalamus, the mind's anxieties can, therefore, stimulate the production of the growth hormones and the growth peptides.

Anxieties probably also increase the receptivity of the cells' membranes for growth hormones, growth peptides or other growth factors.

On a small, but visible scale, it can be seen that anxieties can accelerate the growth of a beard in men, and the nails in both men and women.

Anxieties appear mainly with adolescence and can have an important influence on individual growth, particularly in early adolescence.

Children rarely show a significant difference in their individual height before early adolescence. In early adolescence when the mind starts forming its ego, when the mind starts taking itself too seriously and when the mind starts developing anxieties on a more lasting scale, is when growth differences between individuals become more noticeable.

As my theory that an unhappy adolescence might contribute to the development of the height of an individual, and vice versa, is contrary to many people's expectations, I would like to elaborate on it.

African Pygmies who are the smallest known human adults, are not the smallest when they are children. Pygmy children rank eighteenth in height of 38 ethnic groups. In prepubertal growth there is no significant difference between Pygmies and their non-Pygmy neighbours. It is during their adolescence that Pygmies grow at a lesser rate than other human groups. Research has not found any genetic or cytoplasmic reason for this phenomenon.

I think that this is probably due to the fact that Pygmies are the happiest people in the world. They spend their adolescent and adult lives playing, dancing and giggling in a happy environment. They must have been living for millenia in this way, as we can see Pygmies dancing in the frescos of Egyptian temples depicted some 4,400 years ago.

The daily reality of the Pygmy hunter-gatherers in their tropical forests did not allow for the development of a strongly conceited or pretentious ego that creates anxieties.

Important evidence of the lack of conceit or pretentiousness could be the fact that Pygmies are the least competitive and aggressive of the human groups. Most human competition and aggression is originated and perpetuated by the mind's fantasies and strong beliefs.

Life in a community, where children are all treated the same, without any social hierarchy, prevents the development of envy or jealousy, which carry anxieties.

Pygmies are always very patient and polite, a sure sign of lack of frustration, frustration being a product of the mind's pretentiousness and conceit.

But, one of the most positive evidences that Pygmies are free from anxieties is that they do not suffer from anxiety related diseases such as hypertension, arteriosclerosis, depression or other psychosomatic disorders.

Boys have a more frustrated adolescence then girls. Perhaps, this is why men are taller than women.

Throughout history the aristocracy or ruling classes tended to be taller than the rest of the population. This might have been a result of the idea of superiority that the minds of the ruling class constantly carry. Carrying and coping with an idea of superiority generates anxiety.

Neapolitans consider themselves the cleverest people in the world, which should have made them taller than they are. Their under-average height is probably due to the fact that they spend their adolescence in the loving care and protection of their 'mammas'.

People tend to develop less height in communities with traditions of strong maternal influence.

The young living in large families, with grand-parents around, tend to be average, sometimes under-average, height. With grand-parents around, parents seem to be more parental.

The first born male, particularly in patriarchal communities, tends to be taller than his brothers or sisters. The idea of the responsibility that the first born develops in early adolescence in these communities, and the anxiety that this idea generates can easily contribute to the development of his height.

Developing self-preciousness and pretentiousness, which carry anxieties, an only child can become taller than the average of his community.

The first born child can feel threatened by the appearance of the second child. If this occurs when the first born is in his adolescence, it can influence the development of his height.

Teenagers of some successful parents also tend to develop anxiety's growth. Many parents tend to try and impress their children with their success, which intimidates and confuses children.

Teenagers of selfish, self-centred or divorced parents also tend to develop anxiety's growth.

An anxiety caused by lengthy hospitalisation or a long illness in adolescence can also increase an individual's height.

On average, being more worried than apprentices, students in all countries tend to grow taller than apprentices.

In the Dinaric Alps, along the coast of Dalmatia, people are above average height. Anxiety caused by their precarious economic conditions, might be one of the determining factors of this.
After the First World War many of these mountain people emigrated and settled in Vojvodina, a rich area in the north of Yugoslavia.
Living in better economic conditions, therefore with less anxiety, the descendents of these tall Slavs have now become average height.

In general, people living in polluted and noisy cities are taller than the agricultural population of the same country.

Anxiety, caused by the precarious existence of blacks in the agitated and competitive USA, made them much taller than their brothers in Africa.

Living in a happier and healthier environment, with lesser anxieties than the rest of the population, Australian Aborigines are much smaller than the rest of Australians.

In general terms, individuals living in a caring Socialist Welfare State should tend to be shorter than those living in a restless and competitive Capitalist society.

The height of many Italians noticeably increased with the uncertainty of post-war competitive Capitalism, compared with the Italians who grew up in the more protective corporative economy between the two World Wars.

The Swedish Welfare State, with its tall population might contradict my theory. The depressive loneliness of the Swedish adolescent population, however, could explain their anxiety's growth.

Many claim that improved alimentary and economic conditions over the past century, particularly in the Western World, contributed to the increase of people's average height.

I think one could also, at least partially, attribute this increase to the anxieties brought in the same period by the rapid technological changes, uncertainty, the aesthetic degradation of the environment and to pollution.

Up until a century ago, the average height of most Europeans had remained roughly the same for thousands of years. Since then, the average height started increasing rapidly.

Between 1880 and 1910, a period of increased anxieties, average height increases in the following countries were: France, 1 cm., Italy, 1.1 cm., Switzerland, 2.4 cm., Holland, 3.8 cm., Sweden, 3.1 cm., Japan, 1.5 cm.

Between 1920 and 1960, a period of even more intense anxieties and uncertainties, the average height increased as follows: France, 4.2 cm., Italy, 4.9 cm., Switzerland, 3.6 cm., Holland, 6 cm., Sweden, 4.3 cm., Japan, 6 cm.

Apart from domestic animals, who live in unnatural surroundings, dependent on humans, we are the only creatures able to create superfluous, often damaging extra fat.

There is evidence that anxieties increase our weight, mainly due to the fact that the centres of the appetite and obesity are situated on the hypothalamus, which is highly sensitive to lasting anxieties, frustrations or discontent.

Certain scientists have invented a gene supposed to be responsible for obesity.

This can not explain, however, why an individual with this same gene which kept him fit and slim for years, suddenly, at a certain stage of his life, usually the stage in which anxiety tends to increase, triggers off the production of extra fat.

During and after the middle age crisis, which brings an increase in anxieties, a large percentage of humanity is over-weight.

With the increase in anxieties caused by a new environment, immigrants tend to put on weight.

The breakdown of love-affairs are well known to be the enemies of good figures.

Slim children, on reaching adolescence with its anxieties, often develop extra weight.

The collective anxiety of a community creates the curious impression of a physical similarity among the people of that community, perhaps due to the similarity in their fatness.

There is evidence that obesity is inherited.

In our era dominated by gene mythology, we are informed that this inheritance is due to the inheritance of the obesity gene.

I think that it might be more accurate to say that we also inherit anxieties, or the predisposition for anxieties, experienced by our mother during her pregnancy.

During pregnancy, neuro-transmitters and hormones created in the mothers brain and body by her anxieties, can pass into the embryo, influencing the development of its nervous system and memory, and predisposing the progeny to the anxieties carried by the mother.

Evidence that a mother's emotional arousals influence the child in her uterus is that the child spends a great deal of time dreaming. Without the inherited mother's emotional experiences we could not explain the dreaming of neonates.

Anxiety can drive a number of people to a frantic desire for sugar-based food, all of which is fattening. Perhaps this is triggered off by an urge to escape the anxiety by re-entering their care-free sugar-fed infancy.

Stress

Stress is one of the most discussed subjects of our modern world. Over the past fifty years there have been more papers and books on it than on any other matter, and more and more people attribute the causes of their various afflictions to stress.

What is stress?

As I mentioned before, stress is an extreme range of anxieties.

The difference between anxiety and stress could be explained with alcohol.

Anxiety could be compared to one or two drinks, not necessary harmful, often even beneficial.

Stress can be compared to three drinks or more which can positively damage our physical and mental health.

Moderate amounts of stimulants such as caffeine, theine or nicotine can improve our brain's glandular and mental activities. Stronger doses of these irritants instead produce high blood pressure and heart palpitations which can damage both the body's and the brain's activities.

The passage from anxiety to stress is personal; it can often change in time and space even for the same individual, as do the consequences of the stress.

The difference between anxiety and stress can be seen in the consequences caused by the nervous energies that they generate. Whilst the nervous energy created by anxiety can be useful and beneficial, nervous energy created by stress reduces the efficiency of the brain and the body. For example, an athlete can reach his optimal results under a moderate range of anxieties, but stress can induce muscular stiffness and, in extreme cases, paralysis.

The difference between anxiety and stress is also evident on the stage. With moderate performance anxiety, an actor can achieve the highest levels of his interpretation. With stress, and stress-induced stage fright, however, he can be reduced to clumsiness, rigidity and even speechlessness.

What urges people from one or two drinks to more drinks, from anxiety to stress?

The obvious answer must be the mind's discontent. Most of our reasoning and behaviour is the search for a lesser discomfort, a lesser discontent.

Our mind often tries to solve the problem of anxiety, caused by wishful beliefs or pretentious hopes by escaping into even more wishful beliefs, into even more pretentious hopes.

The escape from anxiety caused by wishful beliefs and pretentious aspirations into capricious beliefs and avaricious or greedy aspirations is what creates stress. The word capricious stems from the Latin 'caput' and 'ericius', meaning hair standing on end – an impression often felt during stress.

Stress is mainly created by our mind and by its excessive pretensions: the more pretentious the mind, therefore, the deeper the threat from reality, the greater the stress.

Many experts talk about stress-agents or the external factors generating stress. In my opinion, it is the mind's responsiveness to these agents rather than the agents themselves which is important. For example, crowded public transport is usually irritating and stressful, whereas much larger crowds at grand social gatherings or pompous receptions seldom bother many people. On the contrary.

People will happily queue for hours to see a famous personality, but queueing for much less time for a bus can induce stress.

In general, due to having more inflated egos and stubborner minds, men are more inclined to suffer from stress than women. Perhaps, this difference explains why, in similar environmental conditions, most women live longer than men. Women who successfully imitate men seem to also succeed in jumping from a life of anxieties to that of stress, and in acquiring the susceptibility to the stress-related disorders and diseases.

As pretentiousness is generated by discontent, and as the mind, by nature, is in permanent discontent as it reflects the constant instability of the brain's cells, the evolution of humans seems to be marching towards ever increasing stress. In fact, we can see a permanent increase in stress-related diseases and mental disorders.
Increasing our pretentiousness and expectations, the continuous cultural, scientific and technological progress seems to being a continuous increase in stress.

It is in the nature of pretentiousness to place itself above an individual's potential to realise its aspirations.
In the search for importance, in our hierarchial society, many people consider it their supreme achievement when they are over-promoted, in other words when they reach a position of incompetence. This makes the stress involved a positive health hazard. Lower down the hierarchical ladder, the stress caused by the resentment of those who fail to be even promoted, is an even worse health hazard.
The continuous increase in our pretentiousness has brought a new form of stress, stress produced by the fast spreading phenomenon called 'underload', when a job is insufficiently challenging, when a job does not fulfil our potential. Given the fact that most people live in a cloud of inflated self-esteem, they also inflate in their minds their potentials.

Most experts underline that hopelessness and despair bring stress and stress-related diseases. They seldom try to find out what caused the hopelessness and despair in the first place. Perhaps, they know that the answer could put the ball into the court of the hopeless and despairing, as their hopelessness and despair are created by their excessive hopefulness and greed.

When by some miracle we achieve our pretensions, we often find further suffering, either because we develop the conceit to deserve more, or we develop a dread that we might lose what we have undeservedly achieved.

Any rational reasoning would see that in its very nature pretentiousness carries self-defeat and failure, but rational reasoning is not in tune with the mind's wishful thinking.

One of the main characteristics of the human species is our ability not only to deceive others, but to deceive ourselves.

Both, self-deceit and deceit increase stress. The former because it is an escape from reality, the latter because it is the falsification of reality aiming at the defence of self-deceit. Most of the time lies and deceits tend to protect self-deceits.

Stresses created by self-deceits or deceits are often visible on people's faces or in their body's rigidity and clumsiness.

Shame, another uniqueness of our species, is an important protection of our physical and mental welfare, as these can be damaged by the excessive stress caused by excessive lies or self-deceits.

Self-deceit and deceit are the instruments used by the self-conceited. Self-conceit leans mainly on the mind's idea that we are able to shape reality in accordance with our wishful fantasies. The mentality that we can shape reality to suit our fantasies creates a permanent challenge and frustration by reality itself.

Many people are convinced that we can win over nature and its reality. This conviction is a result of the insensitiveness of self-conceit. The self-conceited seldom notice the side-effects or consequences of their victories over nature.

In our conceit, we consider ourselves intelligent.

But, are we?

Self-conceit, this creation of the adolescent mentality, is associated with its best ally: cleverness, and cleverness is the negation of intelligence. It is in the nature of cleverness to become an obsession as it has to constantly provide food for self-conceit. Being an obsession, cleverness generates stress, and stress reduces the brain's reasoning to here and now terms, a rushing reasoning. This reasoning consists of taking the maximum advantage of the present, in an unscrupulous exploitation of the moment, without any consideration for the future. The here and now reasoning, dictated by cleverness, has no consideration for the future because it has no past. A reasoning without the past or the future is not an intelligent or wise reasoning.

The worst of the adolescent mentality's self-conceits is its invention of immortality. (Juvenile and mature mentalities are less seduced by the idea of immortality.) All religions preaching the belief of immortality have been successful because their deceit suited the needs of the believers' self conceit.

What is wrong, one might inquire, in believing in immortality?

The wrong is that this belief, like any other belief in the supernatural, creates tension and stress, thereby making the believer's life, and the life of those around him, hell. If we accepted the truth that our life here on this planet is the only life we have, we might be kinder to our neighbours and to our planet.

The second worst self-conceit, particularly of the Western adolescent mentality, is the Judeo-Christian belief that their omnipotent and only God entitled man to be the omnipotent and only ruler of the rest of the natural world.

This wishful belief can only prove itself by going against the natural world and its order. In fact, most Western artistic creations are a tendency towards the domination of nature by either destroying it or brutalising its harmony. Most of Western science is nothing but an aggressive racket againt nature. By unscrupulously exploiting nature, or by denaturalising it, Western mentality's scientists try desperately to prove that they are superior to nature.

Due to the fact that belief carries doubt, belief in superiority or supremacy increases instability. Instability generates action and aggression. Man is never more unstable than when he is wrong. In fact, it is when he is wrong that man is most aggressive. The failure of a believer's aggression leaves him in a deep depression.

We start lying to ourselves and to others with adolescence, when our mind forms its ought to be self, its conceited ego. It is then that we discover the truth about ourselves. In fact, lying aims at hiding or escaping the truth. A child cannot lie. He does not know what the truth is.

As I said before, the difference between a child and an adolescent is while the former plays with his fantasies, the latter takes them overseriously. That is what makes the latter ridiculous. We are proud that we are the only species able to laugh; but, we never point out that we are also the only laughable species. When we laugh at other species, it is because they remind us of our adolescent mentality and its pretentiousness, this source of ridicule. In fact, the pretentious fear humour or derision more than anything.

Self-conceit sometimes places us beyond ridicule, where humour and pathos unite into tenderness. Self-conceit is easily seduced by deceit. It is in the nature of any belief to be attracted by deceits. In fact, all history consists mostly of stories of believers seduced by deceivers.

What makes these stories tender is the fact that believers are not seduced by believers: they are seduced by actors or performers. The most significant leaders in history were all great actors. They all have one important asset in common: a vast store of nervous energy, provided by their performance anxieties.

Pretentiousness implies suffering of the mind, which can be stronger than any physical pain. We are able to put-up with severe pain, and even atrocious physical tortures, to placate the suffering of the mind.

Buddha was wrong to attribute the causes of human suffering to ignorance; he would have done better had he attributed our suffering to pretentiousness, which, in fact, increases when culture and education take over from ignorance, when we start believing that we know things, when we start being conceited. Ignorance implies innocence and humbleness, and these do not cause the mind's suffering or mind-induced stress.

Any increase in pretentiousness increases stress because the higher the aspirations and hopes, the higher the mind's apprehension and dread of their failures. The more the mind is avaricious, the higher is the threat to its existence, the higher the sensation of precariousness, the stronger the activity of the hypothalamus.

With an increase of the activity of the hypothalamus, we have an increase in the activity of the sympathetic nervous system, an increase in the secretion of the adrenaine glands' hormones, and an increase in the emergency-induced secretion of neurotransmitters and of neuropeptides. This brings higher levels of heart activity, blood pressure, and of immunodeficiency. These levels of stress can damage both our physical and mental health.

While anxiety can pass unnoticed, stress is a physical sensation of tension and strain, produced mainly by a contraction of the body's muscles. In fact, the word 'stress' derives from the Latin 'stringere', meaning to tighten, to squeeze.

Over a moderate range of anxieties, our senses, our perception and our reasoning can reach high levels of aliveness and alertness, where with stress they are sensibly reduced, reaching, during extreme stress, total insensitivity and insensibility.

With anxiety we learn as we observe with a wider curiosity. With stress all interest is concentrated on the urgent or immediate survival, and this can also bring us to lose the previous learning.

While a range of moderate anxieties can increase an adolescent's growth to above average, stress can reduce it.

A range of moderate anxieties can prolong life, stress can break it down.

Mild or soft music, and for short periods, can be stimulating, loud music, and for lengthy periods, however, is stressful and damaging.

A moderate range of anxieties can improve productivity in the services and in industry. Stress, instead, reduces this productivity and increases the level of accidents at work.

As I mentioned before, with moderate anxieties our muscular efficiency can reach optimal levels; with stress, efficiency and the control of our muscles are noticeably reduced. In extreme stress we can reach extreme stiffness or immobility.

With certain anxieties eloquence is enriched; with stress it is sensibly reduced. In extreme cases of stress we might resort to violent gesticulation and shouting, or complete rigidity and muteness.

The difference between anxiety and stress is also evident in artistic creativity.

Artistic activity needs energy. An energy can be provided by juvenile exuberance, the adolescent mentality's anxieties, and by maturity's magnanimity or benevolence.

Often the same artist can change his mentality during his life, and with this change, the quality of his art. What a difference, for instance, between Michelangelo's Sistine Chapel's adolescent aggressiveness, compared with the humbleness, magnanimity and eternity of his last work, known as Rondanini Peita. What a difference between Beethoven's heroic style, and the serenity of his last Quartets. Mozart, instead, spent the whole of his life in a playful and exuberate juvenile mentality.

Perhaps, because of these different energies which generate different qualities of art, humanity has never found a unified theory of beauty. It seems that each mentality tends towards its own aesthetic values. The mature mentality finds beauty in grace, elegance, coherence, order or humaneness, all in tune with maturity's serenity. The juvenile mentality might find these values respectful but boring, while the adolescent mentality is often irritated by them. The adolescent mentality might find beauty in brutality or violence, while the juvenile and mature mentalities find brutality or violence ugly and frightening.

The popular saying, 'beauty is in the eye of the beholder' is very accurate. People's aesthetic appreciation relates to their mentalities. A mentality's taste is mainly ruled by its appetite, and an appetite is determined by the mind's needs and their urgency.

A person in need is attracted and seduced by anything that can placate his need. When we are sexually aroused, we can find people attractive that we would not notice if we were not in that state.

While art produced by juvenile exuberance is joyful in its playfulness, and while art created by the energy generated by maturity's benevolence and magnanimity, is calming in its serenity and universality, art realised by the adolescent mentality's anxiety-induced nervous energy can be exciting and exhilarating. Excitement and exhilaration are the result of the intimidating, threatening or aggressive nature of art inspired and realised by anxiety-induced nervous energy. This intimidation can, in some sensitive people, provoke dizziness or sickness.

Medical services, particularly in Italy, are well aware of the Stendhal syndrome. Stendhal was the first person to describe anguish and dizziness during and after visiting an art gallery in Florence. Art created by anxiety creates anxiety in its viewers. This should not be surprising as the main aim of the artistic creation produced by anxiety-induced nervous energy is to impress in order to seduce, seduction being the supreme aspiration of loneliness, this major source of anxieties.

Most Western art is a result of the nervous energy generated by Western people's anxieties. The West is rich in artistic creations because of its richness in anxieties. Periods of history which were filled with anxieties, such as the Fifth century B.C. in Greece, and the Fifteenth and Sixteenth centuries in Italy, were rich in works of art.

Much of the Western geniality and scientific inventiveness is also mostly due to Western people's anxieties, restlessness and agitation.

Many artists or creative geniuses are well known to have long periods of depression. These are usually explained by their inner-emptiness, their lack of creativity.

In my view, this depression is more due to the artist's excessive anxieties or stress, a result of increased pretentiousness. It is not the inner emptiness that causes the depression, but the stress, induced by increased pretentiousness, which creates the sensation of inner-emptiness, the lack of creativity and depression. In fact, this increased pretentiousness can conduce an artist or a genius to mental disorders.

To those who insist that works of art, which are mainly a result of agitation and restlessness, caused by anxiety-induced nervous energy, enoble humans by enriching their souls, I would like to suggest a more accurate study of history in order to discover that many of the worst criminals of our species were either artists or lovers of art. The most violent and brutal eras of history were also rich in artistic creativity and lovers of art.

As far as the adolescent mentality's artist is concerned, there is nothing noble about his artistic creations: he is simply discharging and exteriorising his anxiety-induced nervous energy in a desperate search of importance, so needed by self-importance and pretentiousness.

Women have always been considered way inferior in their artistic or speculative activities by the adolescent mentality.

This should, in fact, be a great compliment to the common sense intelligence and wisdom of women. Given their greater sense of responsibility and their concern with the positive problems of life, women are generally less pretentious and less infatuated than men. Being less pretentious and less infatuated, women have lesser anxiety-induced nervous energy to be discharged in the superfluous.

While stress positively suppresses the body's immune responses, moderate anxieties can enhance immunoefficiency. This is probably due to the fact that the moderate levels of the adrenal glands' hormones, released by moderate anxieties, stimulate the activity of the cells of the body's defenses, while excessive levels of these hormones, caused by excessive anxieties or stress, reduce the activity and efficiency of the cells of the immune system and of the organs generating these cells.

In fact, by reducing the efficiency of the immune system, extra doses of stress-induced hormones, corticosteriods, are used to prevent the rejection of grafted organs by the body's defences.

Stress-related diseases and disorders vary from the common cold to cancer, from headaches to insomnia, from dryness of the skin to that of the mouth, from herpes to nervous twitches, from constipation to diarrhoea, from sweating to fainting, from rheumatoid arthritis to osteoarthritis, from asthma to accelerated breathing, from alergies to multiple sclerosis, from the worry of catching a disease to various forms of mental disorders or suicide.

Stress usually breaks down the body's most vulnerable cells, or most fragile organs. The most vulnerable spot varies from individual to individual, which explains why the same stressful event or condition, such as losing a loved one, causes cancer in some people, an oppotunistic infection in others, a cold or an ulcer in some, arthritis or nothing at all, in others.

The effects of external stressful stimuli, be they nuclear, chemical or biochemical, seem to depend on the pre-existing level of an individual's mind's created stress. Exposed to a cancer causing radition, those who are under high levels of stress, are likely to be more seriously affected.

We all carry certain types of cancer, many kinds of pathogens, and hundreds of various viruses in a dormant state. They remain dormant due to a healthy activity of the body's cells and the efficiency of its immune and repair systems. Any pressure on the cells or any reduction in the efficiency of the body's immune and repair systems can revive one or more of these dormant pathogens or viruses. Every level of an individual's stress carries the reviving power of a disease, related to that level of stress.

Stress can also create what we could call beneficial

diseases. In order to reduce or stop a stressful activity some people make up an imaginary pain or disease, thereby justifying them to reduce their stressful activities.

Present longevity has introduced a new form of stress: the dread, not of getting old, but of looking old. This creates obsessions, such as weight watching, fanatical fitness and all manners of face and body lifting. Any obsession is always stressful.

We also suffer more and more from the dread of becoming ill. We often lose our head in view of some minor or ridiculous signs of unrest or unease.

Being under strong stress, fanatics of any belief or prejudice are also vulnerable to stress-related diseases.

The marginal or oppressed minorities of a collectivity also develop a higher immunodeficiency than the rest of the community.

Some left-handers who feel frustrated because of it, can show a certain deficiency in their natural defenses.

Being stressful, myopia and dyslexia can also reduce the efficiency of the immune system.

The increasing tendency towards professional specialisation, which generates the stressful effects of loneliness, can reduce natural defenses. The increasing division of labour can only expose future humanity to more stress-related diseases.

By reducing team work and togetherness, both in services and industry, thus increasing the feeling of isolation, the introduction of computers is bringing yet another form of stress.

By increasing the alertness and plasticity of the synapses of our brain's cells, a moderate range of anxieties can help us in the consolidation and retrieval of our memories.

Certain moderate doses of anxieties could even be beneficial to brain problems such as senile dementia or Alzheimer disease.

Given the increasing number stricken with this disease, I would like to elaborate my theory.

In order to be able to understand dementia better, I think we should examine how the registration of events in the memory-pool works, and how past experiences are revoked from the memory-pool.

A sensation only becomes a perception after having been scrutinised and valued by our brain. In order to be able to perceive a sensation, our brain must be in a state of perceptiveness.

States of the aliveness and vivacity of our senses and states of the perceptiveness of the brain are dynamic states, states of activity, states of energy.

Each living being is in a fluctuating state of existence, and each state of existence has its own level of awareness and perceptiveness.

What is it that provides the energy needed for the alertness of our senses and the perceptiveness of our brain for openness to new events and readiness for new experiences?

The answer is: mainly the mind's instability, mind-induced anxieties.

Any information perceived by our brain will be registered in our memory-pool on the wave-length of the anxiety it creates, on the frequency of the nervous energy this information produces. In essence, our memories are a network of pathways of the energies left on the brain's cells by different anxieties. The same brain's cells register many memories, all recorded on different intensities of the nervous energy generated by anxieties.

Both rewarding and punishing events, and exciting or inhibiting conditioning, used to facilitate memorisation and learning, in fact, create anxieties without which there would be no memorisation or learning.

That the memory is associated with anxieties can be deduced by the fact that when the emotional centres of our brain (the limbic system) are damaged or inhibited, the registration of new events, or the recollection of past experiences, are considerably reduced.

How are past experiences evoked from our memory?

Events registered in our brain are best revived by the anxiety-induced energies similar in their intensities or frequencies to those which originally encrusted the events.

That the revival of past experiences is provoked by anxieties is best illustrated in dreams. Most dreams take place during REM (Rapid Eye Movement) periods of sleep when the sympathetic nervous system and adrenal glands are noticeably active.

We are not frightened by what we see in our nightmares, we have them because we are in a specific state of anxiety.

One's memory can even be revived by external energy. Electrical stimulation of the brain can revive events which were registered by a similar wavelength of emotional energy.

It is well known that people suffer severe pain in a leg or arm that has been amputated. This usually happens when people experience the same level of anxieties on which these pains were registered in their memory.

Students who did their homework with blaring background music have difficulty remembering what they have learned in the cold silence of a school hall. We revive our learning material better if we acquire the same emotions in which the learning originally took place.

When sober, people have difficulty remembering events which occurred when they were drunk or drugged. Their memory may return, however, when they reach the same state of intoxication.

Deep-sea divers sometimes have difficulty recalling underwater experiences when back on the surface.

Many insist that a 'retrieval clue' can help the access to the memory. This is true, but only when this 'retrieval clue' creates the level of anxieties on which it was previously registered in our memory.

If one learns a foreign language in a concentration camp, for example, one may have difficulty using it in a social or flippant conversation during a dinner party. If the subject of conversation is the war, or depravations, however, which revive anxieties in which the foreign language was learned, the foreign language will be much more fluent.

We do not lose our memory with old age merely due to the reduced efficiency of our brain, but also because in ageing we lose curiosity, and with the loss of curiosity we do not experience the anxieties on which our memories were registered and which can revive them.

This often happens because with age, in search of a more cautious living, the strength of fixed beliefs, of routine reasoning and behaving increases, thereby reducing alertness and curiosity. Increasing with their ageing the strength of their beliefs and of their routine reasoning and behaving, members of religious orders are more susceptible to senile dementia than any other social group.

By reducing curiosity and alertness, boredom, apathy, loneliness or recluseness can also cause dementia. Prisoners serving life sentences or those isolated in solitary confinement tend to develop problems with their memories.

People living in Scandinavian countries, where life is highly organised and more of a routine, have more problems with their memories than people living in the Mediteranean area.

Being more lonely and more role performing, individuals belonging to the middle classes are more susceptible to senile dementia than individuals belonging to working classes.

Scientists claim that the memory of the elderly is weakened by lack of concentration.

But, could it be the contrary?

As part of cautiousness, many old people tend to increase their self-centredness, and this often implies extreme concentration, which reduces the range of curiosity and alertness, limiting the activity of the memory.

By reducing the strength of their fixed beliefs, varying their cliché reasoning or routine behaviour, by trying to avoid loneliness or apathy, by strolling out and about without rushing, the aged could renew their moderate anxieties, therefore their memorisation and their recollection of the past. Sometimes even changing the furniture or pictures around in the home can help to revive mental activity.

Many experts advise old people to stop smoking, to reduce the consumption of coffee, tea or alcohol, because these can damage their health.

I think that we should also take into consideration the fact that many people registered a great deal of their past experiences in their memory-pools when on the levels of anxieties generated by nicotine, caffeine, theine or alcohol.

Obviously, the consumption of these irritants could only help the revival of the past, registered on levels of anxieties caused by these irritants in the past.

Had Proust's doctor told him that carbohydrates or sugars were bad for his health, he would have never experienced 'the taste of the crumb of madeleine soaked in her concoction of lime flowers', which revived emotions and memories of his past, and which memories became the best pages of his artistic creation.

In fact, recently it has been discovered that nicotine, taken in pill form can help those suffering from senile dementia. A pill, however, can never replace the chain of emotions connected with smoking, such as lighting and inhaling a cigarette, cutting and puffing on a cigar and filling, tapping and relighting a pipe.

What is more, taking moderate doses of alcohol, nicotine, caffeine or theine, could also help in another sense. These irritants stimulate the activity of nerve cells and the activity of the nerve growth factors which helps the activity of nerve cells, and this can be beneficial to elderly people's mental activity and memory.

Limiting our emotional experiences, a diminished sensitivity of the cells of our sense organs can sensibly reduce the activity of our memory. In fact, a degeneration of the cells of our smell organ often precedes dementia.

Stress-induced inefficiency of our sense organs dramatically reduces memory's activity.

Some old people resort to a curious defense mechanism against senile dementia: they resort to spontaneity, to liberation from social rules or roles. By liberating themselves from social, and often even moral rules and roles, they start experiencing a variety of emotions and anxieties which help their memory exercises. Some old people start using vulgar or coarse language. Vulgar or coarse language or swearing can, in fact, generate emotional arousals which can revive the memory's activity.

Some old people start a salubrious exercise, that of talking to themselves.

What we lose with age is more the use of memory than the memory itself. With age people can increase their anxieties above a beneficial level, thereby entering the state of stress. Concentrating the brain activity and attention on a here and now interest, stress tends to reduce memorisation and the use of memory to a minimum needed by the immediateness of the moment. During strong stress people are able to escape into partial or total amnesia, sometimes reaching a stage in which they do not even remember who they are.

In extreme stress our perceiving and memory-reviving systems can become paralysed.

Given the importance of stress, I would like to underline once again that stress mainly belongs to the adolescent mentality and its pretensions, overambitions and greed. Stress is not in the nature of juvenile and mature mentalities or in the nature of animals.

The human tragedy, however, is that, being more aggressive than other mentalities, the adolescent mentality is dominating our planet, forcing other human mentalities and animals to live in an atmosphere of stress.

Fatigue

Under pressure, inorganic matter is torn and consumed, resulting in break-down, but organic matter experiences fatigue. Fatigue, however, has an important beneficial effect: it slows down or stops the organism's activity before it is too late, thus enabling it to repair the damage created by the activity. Fatigue induces relaxation and sleep during which the body can recover.

With fatigue the cell's activity noticeably changes. Free radicals, peptides and other molecules which were in a dormant state, revive. Carrying their high biochemical instability, these revived molecules mobilise the activities of the cells in search of their previous state of existence, of their lesser instability, of their dormant state. Perhaps, it is this activity which induces sleep or relaxation. We all notice a deterioration in our alertness, curiosity, perceptivity and reasoning when we are tired or when we did not sleep well, when a different metabolism takes place in our brain's cells.

During the fatigue of an organism, some viruses which were kept in a dormant state inside the cells or inside their nucleic acids, can revive, taking over the organisation of the cells for their reproduction.

Being less selective during fatigue, the cells' receptors become more inviting, allowing pathogens to enter and damage the cells.

Under stress our brain and our adrenal medula release natural opiates which reduce the sensation of fatigue. Preventing the perception of fatigue, stress allows the body to reach an excess in its activity, to reach the point beyond repair. Perception stimulates reaction.

When a person under stress develops the sensation of

fatigue, it is usually too late, as the body's over-activity has already done irreparable damage.

Many of the younger generation of today's hearing is impaired due to loud pop music. The euphoria created by natural opiates, the secretion of which was generated by the stressful noise, prevented the body from feeling any fatigue of the hearing organs at the time.

Stress stiffens the tissues and excessive pressure on stiffened tissues breaks them down.

Frenzied movement and dancing to the beat of loud music is mainly the discharge of nervous energy generated by the irritation caused by frantic music. The noisier the music, the more frenetic the discharge.

Many fights and wars are preceded or accompanied by noisy sounds, to generate the irritation-induced nervous energy needed for fighting.

Loud drums, battle cries or the noise of firing guns can, however, increase the secretion of natural opiates to the point that many soldiers advance towards the enemy forgetting to use their weapons. During the famous offensives in the First World War a third of the soldiers carried their guns without firing.

Opiates releasing chanting is part of religious ecstasy.

After most pop concerts today, the majority of the fans are in such a zombie-like state that they are highly susceptible to accidents. They are also prone to infections because of their reduced immunoefficiency.

Man-made noise, in fact, is a far more damaging factor than we imagine. Recently it has been discovered that underwater noise forces the water population, particularly oceanic mammals such as seals and whales, to abandon noisy areas. Underwater noise also seems to damage fish eggs and reduce the growth fry. Noise also seems to impair these animals' auditory organs, confusing their orientation and reducing the efficiency of their immune systems, exposing them to all manners of infections.

Each individual organism has his own optimal level of fatigue at which he starts reducing the fatigue-causing activity in order to allow recovery. Those who are less sensitive to fatigue, age and break down sooner than those easily tired.

In a multicellular organism, the fatigue of one group of cells spreads over the rest of the body. In fact, the fatigue of one group of cells of an organism starts to reduce the efficiency of the most fragile group of cells, or of the most unstable organ of the body. The organism is like a chain: under pressure the chain breaks down with the breaking down of the weakest link.

It is the most unstable group of cells or the most fragile organ of an organism, in fact, which influences the life of an individual.

As I said, the tendency of an organism is to reach the least possible biochemical discomfort, the least possible instability, with the minimal effort and energy. It is this tendency which might have enabled living matter to acquire learning abilities and memory.

Suffering of the mind tires our nervous centres and their cells, distorting their activities. In fact, it is mainly the fatigue of our nervous centres, and particularly the fatigue of the hypothalamus, which generates stress and stress-related diseases and disorders.

This stress caused by the fatigue of our nervous centres increases with progress. Science and technology may have reduced physical fatigue, but they have noticeably increased the stress caused by the fatigue of our nervous centres. Technology may be replacing physical effort, but the same technology is bringing tension, noise and ugliness, all of which are tiring to our nervous system.

It is in this fatigue of the nervous centres, particularly of the hypothalamus, that we find the typical human afflictions such as nervous break-downs, neuroses, psychoses and suicides.

Fatigue of the hypothalamus can disorganise the activity of the pituitary gland and the activity of the autonomous nervous system. It can also bring radical changes in body temperature, hunger, thirst, water balance, sexual performance, all of which influence our reasoning, our logic and our behaviour.

Above all, fatigue of the hypothalamus can disorganise the secretion of the brain's neurotransmitters which can create depression or other mental disorders.

The following symptoms seem to be connected with mental disorders: pessimism, irritability, intolerance, loss of appetite and sexual potency, insomnia, high blood pressure, palpitations, sweating, pallor, dizziness, malaise, disorientation, aches, migraine, lack of flexibility and reduced efficiency of sense-perception.

These symptoms of mental disorders are basically conditions generated by neuro-endocrine activities during stress.

Most people suffering from some form of mental disorder are also easily offended by any failure in their expectations, which they tend to overdramatise. This overdramatisation increases the suffering of the mind, which increases a disorder in the activity of the hypothalamus and in the activity of other endocrine glands.

Fatigue of the nervous centres can be increased by any activity that we consider an effort, a sacrifice or a humiliation, these being activities which do not please or flatter our inflated ego. The more inflated an individual's ego, the more the activities will be considered an effort, a sacrifice or a humiliation.

There is one safety valve which, with some people, opens at a certain level of their stress. I will call this safety valve stress-induced crying.

Much stress is caused by capricious perseverence in living dangerously in the vacuous gap between pretensions or hopes and the ability to materialise these pretensions or hopes. When our pretensions or hopes suddenly disappear, or when we realise our inability to materialise them or to cope with them, then the stress might disappear. This disappearance often produces relief expressed through crying or sobbing.

Crying and sobbing can be accompanied by laughter when we see that our pretensions or hopes, which had made our life so stressful, were ridiculous or absurd.

Relief through crying can liberate us from our adolescent mentality bringing us either to the playfulness of the juvenile mentality or to the serenity of the mature mentality.

Crying, in fact, is a powerful therapy for any kind of stress.

I would not be suprised if one day scientists discover that the chemical structure of tears produced by stress-induced crying vary from stress to stress. I am sure that through these tears, we eject from the body a certain amount of molecules that kept our body under stress. That is, perhaps, why we usually feel better after a good cry.

In fact, recent research has revealed that emotional tears or tears induced by stress contain 25% more proteins than tears provoked by the external irritation of the lacrimal glands.

Pain

Pain is another significant factor in the survival strategy. It is a signal of danger to the body for it to deal with the causes of the pain before irreparable damage occurs.

Increasing the secretion of natural opiates, or natural painkillers, stress decreases sensitivity to painful stimuli. (The natural opiates bind to pain receptors and so block the sensors of pain).

Extreme stress, caused by extreme suffering of the mind, can produce total insensitivity to pain. We can continue fighting in a stressful battle, or we can continue competing in an agonistic game, even when seriously wounded. By not feeling the pain of the wound, the continuation of the battle or struggle can, however, aggravate the wound, producing irreparable consequences to the body. With the feeling of pain, we would try to eliminate the cause of it before it is too late.

It could be that life itself carries pain, that life is nothing by prolonged painful tension. The high instability which characterises the order of life implies a biochemical discomfort, and this must imply strain or pain. The general tendency of living molecules to move towards a lesser discomfort would have never taken place if the biochemical discomfort was not painful.

Perhaps, due to the natural painkillers released by the living matter and its nervous systems, we do not feel the pain of life, except in moments when the pain crosses a certain threshold, the moments when pain becomes superior to the analgesic effect of the natural endorphins and enkephalins.

The reduction of the responsiveness to the pain realised by acupuncture is probably due to the fact that stress and tension caused by the irritation of the sensitive parts of the body by the needles, produce an extra secretion of natural opiates.

Believing in the efficiency of acupuncture, coupled with the dread that we might be proved wrong in our belief, creates a kind of a self-induced analgesia which contributes to acupuncture efficiency.

Even vaginal irritation, and the pressure or irritation of any other sensitive part of the body can also generate a stress-induced analgesia.

It is a known fact that animals and humans can become insensitive to pain stimuli during sexual arousals. This is probably due to the presence of an extra quantity of natural opiates in the body, the secretion of which is stimulated by the irritating sex cells.

Many trendy shops and boutiques, especially those catering for unstable teenagers, play loud music. Generating stress-induced natural opiates, this noise often pushes the customers into euphoric buying. Influencing rationality, this racket in these shops ought to be banned.

Stress-Addiction

Slowly on we are turning into stress-addicts: we are becoming more and more hooked on our own opiates. Stress is our drug-pusher, the provider of our natural opiates. Like drug-addicts, stress-addicts have their withdrawal symptoms when the stress is over.

We seem to thrive on complaining, dramatising or catastrophising most of the time. We seem to enjoy suffering for problems which are often laughable. We are more and more fascinated or thrilled by disasters. Perhaps, this is why the media emphasises bad news much more than good. Even our entertainment is becoming more stressful, consisting mainly of raucous deafening music, of laments, or of dramas dealing with brutality, crime and violence.

Adventure and taking risks is a breath of life to many. They provide excitement or euphoria because they provide the stress-induced natural opiates. Most braveries, like many other irrationalities, in fact, usually take place in a state of excitement or euphoria generated by stress-induced natural opiates.

Excitement or euphoria, experienced by pilots during their first flights, is caused by the extra secretion of natural opiates which are provided by the feeling of precariousness of being above the laws of gravity, and by the apprehension that things could go wrong. For many, in fact, flying is an addiction.

Providing similar excitement or exhilaration, stress-inducing robbery, rape, vandalism, hooliganism, violence, illegality, rebellion, gambling, expeditions, travelling and overspeeding can also become addictions.

Only a mind-induced stress-addiction could explain the typically human phenomenon, workaholism. By now, stress has become a status symbol for many businessmen.

Only stress-addiction could have inspired the idea of guilt. Perhaps guilt was supposed to have a similar function as physical pain, as physical pain reminds us to take care of our bodies, guilt is supposed to remind the mind to take care of its moral sanity. The mind, however, discovered pleasure in suffering. Perhaps, this is why it invented the idea of 'original sin'.

Could it not be that homosexuality, which belongs to the adolescent mentality, is the result of natural opiate addiction?

Some adolescents find that by assuming an attitude contrary to the established social values or by challenging the natural order, which generates stress, gives them a 'high'.

That homosexuality is a stressful state of existence can be deduced by the fact that the efficiency of many homosexuals' immune systems is below average, thereby exposing them to all kinds of opportunistic infections.

Hormonal changes in homosexuals can be explained by the power of the mind's attitudes and fantasies to influence the activity of the body's endocrine glands, particularly the secretion of the hormones regulating our sexual arousals and our sexual preferences.

Rushing, this characteristic of the West and Japan, which is as irrational as it is dangerous, could only be explained as a stress-induced intoxication. Rushing, in fact, considerably reduces our sensitivity and perceptivity.

Rushing, this absurdity created by the big and complex human brain, the latest achievement in evolution, contributes to the validity of my general thesis that life, from protozoa to Homo sapiens, is a continuous escape from a biochemical discomfort towards a lesser one, from the mind's discontent to a lesser one. Rushing is an escape from discontent. The more discontented we are, the more agitated we are and the more agitated we are the more we rush.

It is interesting to observe the frantic rush which takes place in Western countries the few weeks preceeding X-mas. Becoming part of a big festivity increases our sense of self-importance, which increases our expectations and pretentiousness, and this increases the agitation and rush which implies insensitivity, therefore, rudeness and vulgarity. This pre-X-mas increase in self-importance and agitation is often paid for by many with post-X-mas suicidal depression and opportunistic infections.

Another date around which many individuals increase their sense of self-importance, therefore their agitation and restlessness, is their birthdays. In fact, serious changes in many people's lives seem to take place around that date.

Working with refugees in Italy, it was interesting to note that many of them had escaped their country of origin around their birthday or a few days before or after the date of their national festivity.

Stress-induced natural opiates could explain Jewish reluctance to assimilate with the population of the country they have lived in for generations. To persevere in being different is always stress-inducing.

The irrationality of chauvinism, together with the irrationality of other prejudices, can only be explained by stress-induced excitement. Living with any prejudice is stressful as it places us on the brink of precariousness.

The Nazi's idea of superman generated powerful stress. In fact, many Nazi crimes were committed in a kind of drugged state, under the influence of stress-induced opiates.

Only stress-induced excitement or euphoria could have produced such unnecessary and destructive revolutions.

Stress-induced opiates could explain the pleasurable sensations of the many dangerous sports, such as mountain climbing or motor racing.

Stress-induced opiates could explain the excess, often health damaging, in physical excercises.

Stress-induced natural opiates could explain the excitement of going abroad, particularly for the first time. Facing the unknown or imponderable is stressful, therefore creating the biochemical conditions of excitement.

Only stress-induced excitement provided by the challenge of the natural order and the provocation of its laws can explain the increasing obsession with genetic manipulation. Under stress, our reasoning is reduced to a here and now, regardless of the consequences.

Our complacency towards the polution of our planet can only be explained by stress-induced indolence. Living with polution is stressful.

Our acceptance of the increasing ugliness of the environment, and our unscrupulous exploitation and waste of natural resources can only be explained by stress-induced intoxication. Ugliness is intimidating, therefore stressful.

Many religious or spiritual leaders, moral teachers or gurus, as well as many charlatans, give some advises on how to reach a 'state of blissfulness'. These leaders, teachers or charlatans insist that bliss is the supreme achievement, as in blissfulness we reach blessedness which is an intimate hug from an imaginary divinity.

Blissfulness and despair are intimately related, as the latter generates the natural opiates which create the former.

Despair of the suicidal, despair caused by terminal disease, despair of those who have lost everything, despair caused by a natural catastrophe, are all capable of providing a state of blissfulness.

The Christian God promises grace, on condition that you fear Him. Stressful fear, in fact, is able to stimulate a secretion of endorphins and enkephalins.

We all proudly revel in romantic love and the bliss it provides. But romantic love only provides bliss because it brings despair, the despair of losing the loved one and being forced into isolation and loneliness. Hence the expression: 'we are desperately in love'. In fact, those who are more fragile and those scared of loneliness are always more romantic and more desperate in their loves. Romantic love, as such, is taken far less dramatically by those who belong to tribes, communities or big families. Romantic love prospers more in the Western world than in any other part of the globe.

Mind-induced euphoria must have given us the idea to indulge in external opiates or drugs. The receptors of our brain cells for naturally secreted opiates became the receptors for all manners of man-made drugs to either replace or increase the effect of natural opiates.

More and more adolescents, particularly those who are capricious in their adolescent mentality, are becoming drug addicts. There is a tendency to justify these drugs-takers or addicts with the excuse that they need to escape the 'cruel reality'. Reality is always cruel for those with excessive self-infatuation or pretentiousness. Most drug-addicts seem to be offended by the very existence of reality.

If stress continues to increase with progress, then our species might disappear one day in an agonising euphoria.

Individuality

Stress-induced drug addiction must have added to human individuality, a cult which implies a lonely and isolated existence, nonsensical for such a social species. The only explanation for this nonsensical phenomenon of human individuality must be found in the fact that the stressful life of lonely and isolated individuals is an important source of brain-produced opiates.

In its constant discontent, the human mind discovered that by challenging nature it can induce the secretion of natural opiates which provide a drugged existence, an existence of excitement, exhilaration, euphoria or ecstasy.

The main sign of increased insecurity and vulnerability in the isolated individual is the increase in the isolated individual's selfishness and self-centredness. Any increase in an individual's insecurity or precariousness carries an increase in selfishness and self-centredness, unscrupulousness and ruthlessness, cruelty and violence. Any increase in an individual's insecurity and precariousness also carries a reduction in the efficiency of the senses and perception, and analytical or ponderous reasoning.

What is more, our cult of individuality and our glorification of individual freedom, this pillar of individuality, must be the product of a mental activity under the influence of brain-produced opiates, which opiates have been generated by the stress caused by the individual's precarious existence in his isolation and loneliness.

Like any other idealisation, the idealisation of individuality increases anxieties and stresses to the point of mental disorder.

The cult and glorification of individuality and individual freedom could be classed as mental disorders because they increase an individual's selfishness, self-centredness, rigidity, insensitivity, all the main characteristics of mental disorders. In extreme cases of loneliness, hallucinations can develop.

The effect of natural opiates released under stress by loneliness, can be detected in moments when one reaches a higher degree of individual freedom. The increased precariousness created by the increase in individual freedom can bring exhilaration.

By fleeing to a desert or some other remote corner of the globe, an individual can achieve total freedom, which carries extreme precariousness. This extreme precariousness can produce euphoria or ecstasy, in which supernatural revelations or messages are perceived.

At some level of individual freedom, an individual can reach a certain loneliness in which he finds the beatitude of a narcissist when he is annihilated by his image.

It seems that people with the adolescent mentality escape into individuality and individual freedom in order to aleviate or to placate, with the stress-induced opiates that individuality and individual freedom provide, the tension and biochemical discomfort caused by the increased activity of the body's sympathetic nervous system and of the increased activity of the body's glands that take place in an emergency, brought on by the adolescent rebelious mentality.

People belonging to juvenile and mature mentalities seldom feel the need to escape into individuality and individual freedom because of their lesser biological discomfort which is due to a more harmonious activity of the autonomous nervous system and to a more balanced activity of the endocrine glands.

There is an increasing number of individuals who irritate or offend friends, relatives or authority to the point of being rejected or alientated in order to enjoy their drugged state caused by solitude or loneliness.

Individual freedom is an escape from natural responsibilities and social obligations. Being an escape, individual freedom carries a range of anxieties, from moderate anxieties to stress: the higher the individual freedom, the higher the anxieties. The higher the anxieties, the more selfish and the more self-centred an individual becomes. The more selfish and the more self-centred an individual becomes, the more precarious is his existence, the more restricted his mental activity. In this restricted mental activity, an individual can not realise the paradox consisting of the fact that in the stress caused by the precariousness or panic of a lonely existence there is no individual freedom.

In his self-deceit, produced probably by the activity of the brain under the influence of stress-induced opiates, the human individual has invented a wishful idea, that of individual free will. An individual has only one freedom in his life and this is to end his life. But, even this is an escape.

A major aspiration of the alienated and lonely individual is self-confidence, and this isolates the lonely even more.

Self-confidence does not exist in nature. It is a wishfulness created by a lonely individual's mind. In fact, it is the anxiety which is inherent in any wishfulness that provides self-confidence with energy.

An excessive wishfulness, which transforms self-confidence into excessive self-confidence or stubborness can reduce alertness, curiosity, communicability, togetherness, a sense of reality and prudence enough to expose the self-confident to all manners of accidents. The extreme self-confidence of an ardent believer can reach a stress produced drugged state of euphoria or ecstasy.

Being more humble by nature, juvenile and mature mentalities seldom assume an attitude of self-confidence.

By limiting mental activity and reasoning, self-confidence is a major source of crime and violence.

For years it was fashionable to explain that economic depravation was the main source of crime and violence. I think that economic prosperity is often more responsible for crime and violence than economic misery. More crime and violence are committed on a full stomach than on an empty one. In fact, crime and violence have increased with economic prosperity and progress. With the increase of economic prosperity and progress, self-confidence and self-righteousness increase, without which there is no crime or violence.

Causing stress, therefore generating the secretion of extra natural opiates, strong self-confidence can commit crimes and violence in an exhalted or even a euphoric state. It is not so much the alcohol which makes British hooligans vandals abroad, it is also the excitement caused by the extra secretion of natural opiates. They are drugged by their self-confidence inspired by their wishful belief of superiority at being British.

It is not really surprising that crime and violence belong to the world of the mind. After all, the supreme aim of the mind, its very reason for existence, is to break with nature and its laws, or force them to adapt to the supernatural world created by the mind and its inflated and righteous ego.

The main sources of crime and violence are hostility, hatred, rivalry, vindictiveness, envy or jealousy, all of which are creations of the mind and its inflated ego. A rapist is not a sexual maniac, he is an egomaniac. Aggressive and violent militancy, as well as cruel tortures, are mainly committed by self-confident believers, often in a self-induced drugged state.

That self-confidence is not part of nature but a wishful creation of the mind can be seen from the fact that when it fails, it becomes ridiculous. The truth in nature can always be recognised, as, whatever happens to it, it is never ridiculous or laughable.

By increasing individuality and the individual's self-confidence, the increase in economic prosperity increases people's rudeness, impoliteness and unfriendliness. The French used to be more 'courtois', the English more lady-like and gentlemanly, the Americans kinder, and the Italians more humane before they achieved their higher standards of living.

This can be explained by pointing out that each step up the ladder of economic progress increases instability, therefore forces anxiety more and more towards levels of stress. The pursuit of wealth is the pursuit of stress.

At levels of high anxieties our brain's mental activity is reduced to the unscrupulous 'here and now', or to the short term violent either/or way of reasoning and behaving.

With economic progress many working-class people start assuming the attitude of the adolescent middle-class mentality, to keep up with the Joneses', which brings working-class people towards an increase in selfishness, self-centredness, greed, anxiety and stress, often resulting in unemployment.

The reduced reasoning of the self-confident is best seen when self-confidence reaches levels of heroism, the mind's capricious, often suicidal, challenge to reality.

There is nothing noble in heroism. In reality a hero is seldom after his heroic deeds, he is simply trying to escape from an unbearable anxiety. Heroism often consists of helplessness trying to help hopelessness.

When a heroic act is an escape from deep stress, the hero is often left in a euphoric state, created by the opiates generated by that stress. In fact, a hero often only realises his heroic deeds after the effects of the opiates have subsided, when, in a more sober state, he is congratulated by others.

We are attracted by precipices because, in our panicky way of reasoning when, at the edge of a precipice, we find that jumping off it is the best way to escape the high anxiety caused by the precariousness we feel at its edge.

Any increase in the individual's sense of self-importance can increase his self-confidence. In fact, needing to force those they lead towards certain irrational or heroic deeds, political or military leaders start by flattering their followers' egos, thus increasing the self-conceit and self-importance in them.

Many scientists insist that there is a neurological explanation for our behaviour. They omit to explain, however, what it is that triggers off the hormones and neurotransmitters which are at the basis of the biology of the behaviour.

As the level of the testosterone hormone in the blood of those with self-confidence and with pathological behaviour is higher than normal, many conclude that testosterone must be the hormone of abnormal behaviour and aggression.

We might have a clearer picture of the biology of behaviour, however, if we explained that the extra secretion of testosterone is a result of a specific state in the brain's glandular activity, and that the brain's glandular activity can be manipulated by the mind, by mental attitudes. An ego-flattering prejudice or a wishful belief can inspire self-confidence and aggression because they trigger off the secretion of an extra quantity of aggressive hormones and neurotransmitters.

There is an established conviction that the quest for more and more individual freedom is in human nature.

But, is it?

In reality the quest for more and more individual freedom must be a result of the restlessness and agitation of the adolescent mentality. There is no such quest with juvenile and mature mentalities: they both need community, the former for belonging and protection without which its playfulness could not take place, the latter for its benevolence and prodigality.

There is no freedom in nature: nature is ruled by the laws of nature. Individual freedom, therefore, can only be realised at the expense of nature and its laws. In fact, the adolescent mentality's notion of freedom is on this line. Freedom is always an escape from law and order. That is what makes individuality and its freedom stressful states of existence.

That individual freedom is not in accordance with nature is evident from the fact that it has to be politically or judicially guaranteed and enforced. Rights need laws.

What is more, individual rights generate self-righteousness, and this is a major source of nastiness, ugliness and aggression in life.

Further evience that individual freedom is not in accordance with nature is that any increase in individual freedom increases restlessness and agitation which can result in panic. Any increase in individual freedom also increases anxieties and stresses which can reduce the efficiency of the immune system. Countries with higher individual freedom have a higher rate of psychosomatic disorders.

That individuality and its freedom are an escape into the wishfulness of our mind is evident in moments when a positive fear, such as war or a natural catastrophe, take place. Eliminating the mind's wishful abstractions, poses and affectations, a positive fear eliminates individuality and its freedom, uniting people into a community, an intimacy and togetherness, often embracing total strangers.

That individuality and its freedom are creations of the wishful mind can be seen from the fact that they can become passions and obsessions.

That individuality and individual freedom are creations of the mind can be seen from the fact that the energy that their practice needs is provided by the mind's created anxiety and its nervous energy.

We pay dearly for our quest for individual freedom when old age approaches, when we start developing the most stressful vision, that of dying in loneliness, in an anonymous hospital ward, far from community, family and friends, eliminated by our individuality and its freedom. We also visualise ourselves passing into total oblivion after death, and this can become a nightmare, a nightmare which can accelerate death.

People living in a community, in an extended family, or in the mature mentality take the thought of death less dramatically.

Some political systems promise lasting contentment by realising a stable and rigid social and economic order. After a certain pause in an orderly and rigid political system, people start fighting for more and more individual freedom. Discontent is inherent in the human mind, and a discontented mind craves opiates.

The lonely individuals tried to placate the anxiety of their precarious existences through a novelty in nature: private property.

Leaning on private property, the lonely individual hoped to give a realistic basis to individual freedom, and to reduce the anxiety that his loneliness carried. The contrary happened: the proprietor became a slave of his property; he developed dread of losing it, of being robbed of it, or that it might lose its value. It is inherent in private property to be enclosed, protected and defended. Private property creates the idea of public property, an enemy, an antagonist to fight. The idea of 'mine' creates the idea of 'ours', the former dreading the latter. In fact, when the lonely adolescent mentality individuals came to power they introduced Draconian punishments against the violation of private property. Victorian Britain, in which private property and individual wealth were sacrosanct, used to punish crime against private property and an individual's wealth, most severely.

As each new anxiety has its own brain's glandular activity and its own reasoning and logic, anxiety created by the institution of private property created its own philosophy, morality, economy and culture.

People defending capitalism insist that private property is the major factor in an individual's economic productivity.

This is true. Private property increases an individual's economic productivity because it increases the individual's anxiety, an anxiety which generates a great deal of nervous energy, restlessness, agitation, adventurousness, mobility and aggression. All of these are essential factors of capitalist economy and its efficiency.

Stress caused by isolation and loneliness created another novelty in nature: greediness.

Taken in the sense of an obsessive desire for more and more wealth and possessons, greediness can reach in cupidity the proportions of mental disorder.

Stress-induced opiates could play a significant role in shaking our neo-cortex and our limbic system so much as to place us under the influence of our predatory and rapacious reptilian legacy.

Stress caused by isolation and loneliness can also generate greed for food, which in obesity can reach danger levels to both health and mind.

This disorder can even reach levels of voraciousness when, shaken by the opiates, our brain becomes influenced by our reptilian heritage.

What is more, stress-induced opiates not only influence the quantity of food an insatiable consumes, but also his preference for food that contains substances that help or stimulate the natural opiates.

Even those who are not greedy by nature tend to increase their food intake during stress, manifesting a preference for specific food.

Stress-induced opiates could also play a significant part in anorexia nervosa. There is, in fact, an increase above normal in the amount of opiates in the brain of anorexic girls.

Perhaps, having to cope with adolescence, coupled with wanting to look their best, teenage girls discover the relief, or even the pleasure, in the drugged existence created by stress-induced opiates.

Besides, hunger, which is well known to increase the brain opiates, and which started as a means of keeping the body in shape, in reality, becomes a way of increasing and perpetuating the drugged state in which these girls find refuge from a world which is unsympathetic to their excessive self-centredness.

The cult of individuality started establishing itself firmly in Ancient Greece and became an important factor of Western culture, politics and economy with the Renaissance.

With the rise of cities and of urban life, which meant the rise of the middle-class, the cult of individuality and the glorification of individual freedom rose progressively.

Cities and the urban culture and style of life were formed and kept alive mainly by the bourgeoisie or the middle-classes. The middle-class was formed by rootless, lonely, alienated or self-alienated adolescent mentality individuals. These lonely adolescent individuals gave the main characteristics to the middle-classes all around the world. These characteristics were, and are: excessive selfishness and self-interest, self-assertion, restlessness and agitation, and cleverness or craftiness, based on unscrupulous exploitation and profit-obsession.

What I call the middle-class would mean more a middle-class mentality that the middle-class in to-day's social, political or economic sense. In fact, one can find individuals of the middle-class mentality in all social classes.

The middle-class replaced the intimacy, togetherness and sociability of our species with cool privacy and intimidating secrecy.

The middle-class produced its own hero, Machiavelli, who placed the main characteristics of the narrow and shallow reasoning of the lonely individuals on a pedestal of virtues. These were unscrupulous selfishness and cynical opportunism, which became the main component of cleverness, meaning craftiness, expedience, and trickery. In the eyes of the middle-class, cleverness became superior to intelligence. This belief is in tune with the narrow and shallow short term reptilian way of reasoning created by the stress of loneliness.

The rise of the cities with their anonymous way of life, increased individual isolation and loneliness which increased the cult of individuality even more.

The increase in the middle-class cult of individuality increased anxiety. This increased anxiety increased the individuals' nervous energies. These increased nervous energies increased restlessness, agitation and aggression which helped the middle-class on its way to political and economic power. Conquering power, the middle-classes acquired even more nervous energy by developing the anxiety of those who dread losing the acquired power.

The rise of the middle-classes in Northern Europe produced Protestantism, a direct contact between the individual and his omnipotent God. The Protestant middle-classes separated from Rome much more because of the Catholic Church's Canon Law's restrictions on the exorbitant interest rate on loans, than because of faith.

The cult and practice of individuality reached its glorious period in the Western World in the seventeenth and eighteenth centuries. During this period, known as 'Enlightenment', the lonely individual's characteristics, like unscrupulous selfishness and excessive self-interest, became an individual's 'natural laws'. These natural laws were a part of the 'immutable laws of the Universe.' What is more, an individual's selfishness and self-interest were proclaimed to be in the public interest.

In their excitement, generated by the precariousness caused by their pretensions, leaders of the Enlightenment saw the future as a 'General progress of mankind towards perfection.'

Leaders of the Enlightenment might, perhaps, be less euphoric about the progress of mankind if they could see the continuous increase in people believing and being guided by fortune-tellers, horoscopes, superstition, psychoanalysis or by charlatans.

Excited by stress-induced opiates, the French middle-class committed one of the greatest absurdities in history: the French Revolution of 1789. In their stress-induced euphoria, the French middle-classes did not even notice the ridicule of the fact that when on that glorious day of 14 July 1789 they organised their dramatic assault on the Bastille, in order to liberate the 'oppressed'. They found three lunatics and an ordinary thief. They were liberated!

It is curious to note that many historians insist that with the French Revolution the modern era of history began.

In their excitement, French revolutionary leaders produced the 'Declaration of the Rights of Man'. This declaration, in essence, became a guide helping the individual to reach higher individuality, higher isolation, and deeper loneliness.

The French middle-class proclaimed their great principles of the Revolution: Freedom, Equality, Fraternity.

In their way of reasoning, restricted by stress-induced euphoria, the 'citoyens' and 'citoyennes' of France did not realise that these principles contradicted each other. Freedom can not coexist with equality or fraternity. Equality kills freedom and fraternity, and fraternity negates freedom and equality.

What is more, each individual mind has its own wishful idea of liberty, its own wishful idea of equality, its own wishful idea of fraternity.

Perhaps, this explains why the French middle-class is so passionately litigious.

The middle-class created its own State: nation-State, nationalistic or patriotic State. Being based on wishful prejudices of national superiority, patriotism generates anxiety and anxiety's nervous energy. This nervous energy contributed a great deal to the nationalistic or imperialistic wars of the nineteenth century, and to another absurdity of history: the First World War.

To an impartial, detached mature observer, the First World War must have given the impression that European political leaders and their masses were in a state of intoxication, drugged by the stress-induced opiates, produced by the prejudices of national superiorities.

A Cannibal war correspondent reported the following message to his newspaper: 'Here people kill each other, but they do not eat each other!' was the joke of a French humourist during that war.

The madness which took place during the First World War must have proved without doubt that either there is something wrong with the human new brain, the volume of which we are so proud, or that the natural opiates produced in the brains of lonely individuals, full of wishful prejudices, are able to confuse the human neo-cortex, thus reducing its reasoning efficiency.

With their brains, fuddled by their brains' opiates, Western European missionaries did not find their westernisation of Africa ridiculous. To those African peoples, living in harmony with nature, Western missionaries gave their restlessness, agitation, arrogance, aggression, psychosomatic diseases and mental disorders.

Establishing itself in the Western World, the lonely middle-class mentality introduced its values in all fields of life, from philosophy to science, from economy to ethics.

Western philosophy is the product of the brain activity of lonely individuals under pressure of the mind's created anxiety. Western dialectic consists of a thesis fighting an antithesis in order to reach a synthesis, which instantly becomes a thesis, which continues to fight its antithesis, and so on. This implies a state of hostility and intollerance, a state in which 'who is not with me is against me', a state of persecution, aggression, crime and violence.

I will explain later that this kind of reasoning is much more in tune with our reptilian legacy than with the reasoning of our mammalian brain, our more sociable and more tolerant limbic system, or with our more understanding and broader operating new brain. It seems that our mental activity becomes dominated by our reptilian heritage when our limbic brain and our neo-cortex are shaken in the efficiency of their activities by the brain-produced opiates, secreted under stress, inherent in the precariousness and uncertainty of loneliness, particularly in that extreme precariousness and uncertainty that the loneliness of pretentious philosophers carry.

The reptilian brain implies a short term reasoning, the here and now behaviour, an instant gratification of ruthless selfishness and unscrupulous self-centred cleverness.

The greater our adolescent individuality and individual isolation are, the more our reasoning and behaviour would be influenced by our reptilian brain.

Western science is mainly a middle-class mentality's science, an arrogant and aggressive science, aiming at dominating, exploiting and denaturalising nature.

The mental attitude that we are superior to nature, limits our possibilities to reach the truth. In the adolescent middle-class way of reasoning the truth is mainly victim of the mind's prejudices or beliefs, of the mind's attitude.

The best example of the adolescent mentality's wishful attitude ignoring the truth in the name of its own wishful 'truth' is the centuries lasting insistance that our planet was the centre of the universe around which the sun and the rest of the universe was going around. Until the sixteenth century it was dangerous to think differently.

In Ancient Greece, some mature mentality observers discovered that our planet is only a small part of the universe and, like the rest of the planets, circulated around the sun.

Being caused by restlessness and agitation, a great deal of Western science is unnecessary or superfluous. Most of our scientists, in fact, are not inspired or guided by the realistic needs of humanity in their research, but by their restlessness caused by the needs of their inflated egos, or by their obsessive aspiration to gain the Nobel Prize.

In fact, we have more beneficiary results from the scientific explorations of juvenile and mature mentalities than from the exploiting adolescent mentality's approach.

The juvenile mentality's playful exploration, guided by the trial and error method, unearthed a great deal of our common sense knowledge and of our useful inventions.

Inspired by its more universal attitude, by viewing life as a whole, the mature mentality's science provides a more wholistic, therefore, a more beneficiary knowledge.

Being a mentality of an isolated and a lonely individual, the adolescent middle-class mentality tend to lean on reductionism, which consists of a hope to explain complex phenomena through their isolated individual components.

With the increase of the cult of individuality and individual freedom even religions and ideologies tend to be less and less universal and more and more personal.

The adolescent mentality scientist has difficulty in using the experimental method of trial and error in his research. The more his ego is inflated, the less he will realise he has erred, instead the more he will persevere in his error, often glorifying it.

The adolescent mentality has what could be called witness syndrome or the participant's magnification or valorisation of a witnessed event. Witnessing an event, an inflated ego considers that event important. The more conceited an ego, the more important and the more magnified the event he witnessed. Perhaps this is why it is so difficult for the adolescent mentality to recognise it has erred, which in the search for truth is of capital importance.

Many scientists insist that scientific truth can be unearthed by establishing hypothesis and then by aiming to scrutinise it, or to criticize it, trying to prove it wrong.

Most of the time the adolescent middle-class mentality becomes obsessed with its ideas. The creator tends to fall in love with its creation. Falling in love reduces our sensitivity towards reality.

The worry or anxiety that his hypothesis might be wrong, reduces the efficiency of the sense/perception and reasoning of the scientist, often to the point of ignoring or rejecting whatever might prove him wrong.

How his mentality can influence a scientist's work is best seen in Darwinism. Darwin's theory of evolution through natural selection and the survival of the fittest, could have only been developed in a world dominated by the arrogant, aggressive, unscrupulous and selfish middle-class mentality individuals, a world of the successful and victorious Victorian Great Britain. Social Darwinism was already ruling Great Britain when Darwin announced his theory. Adam Smith preceded Darwin.

Adam Smith's theories in economy were based on the individual struggle, on individual selfishness and self-interest, on individual aggression and on his exploitation based on his personal profit-motive.

Evolution based on natural selection seems to work backwards, as far as our species is concerned, dominated by isolated individuals, operating in an isolated system.

It seems that we only have a chance of survival, a chance to compete with other unscrupulous and selfish individuals if we are even more self-confident, more aggressive, more unscrupulous, more selfish, more cruel in exploitation than they are.

In order to be all that, in order to be more successful than others, we must then eliminate intelligence and the wise pondering of the neo-cortex, abandon the humaneness and sociability of the limbic system, and allow our brain's activity and our behaviour to be dominated as much as possible by our reptilian legacy.

But could it not be that reliance on our reptilian heritage is mainly due to the unreliability of our big brain because of its complexity brought with the increase in its volume. In fact, in serious or mortal danger, most humans forget to use the analitical power of the new brain and the humaneness and sociability or emotions of the limbic system, and follow a behaviour dictated with impulsive immediacy by the reptilian brain.

Or, could it be that in mortal danger we become guided by the reptilian brain's influence because our new brain's efficiency is too shaken by the stress-induced opiates generated by the individual's individuality and its inflated ego.

Western science is obsessed with laws. This is probably due to the influence of Judeo-Christianity and its obsession for eternal laws, an absurdity in the world of uncertainty.

Inspired by a more universal attitude, by looking at life and the cosmos less self-centredly, therefore, less wishfully, the mature mentality discovered the elementary truth centuries ago, a truth ignored by the agitated and pretentious adolescent mentality. This elementary truth simply explains that the essence of life and the essence of the universe, in its expansion or contraction, is made up of instability and uncertainty. Universal instability and uncertainty are reflected in the human mind's permanent discontent.

Given this simple truth that no human agitation or pretentiousness can ever eliminate the mind's discontent, we are only left with one choice: that of trying to placate this discontent. We can only placate the mind's discontent through humbleness, humaneness and humour, by shaking or by deriding our inflated egos. In fact, we could have a safer survival and a more intelligent or pleasant life with just one of these mental attitudes: humbleness implies humaneness and humour, humaneness implies humbleness and humour, and humour implies the other two.

Many religions preach humbleness.

Due to the tension and anxiety that belief inevitably carries, because of the doubt involved, an ardent believer can seldom be spontaneously humble. He is then forced to pretend to be humble, and feigned humbleness is either ridiculous or aggressive.

The lonely individuals of the middle-class mentality developed their main economic theory: capitalism.

The communists accuse capitalism of alientating the people, but, in reality, it is alienated individuals who created, and keep capitalism alive.

Capitalists insist that capitalism is more productive than any other economic system. This is because individuality, individual freedom, private property and the cult of unscrupulous cleverness create much anxiety, and this generates a great deal of the nervous energy which provides capitalism with its economic productivity.

Audacity, aggressiveness, risk-taking and adventurousness are all inspired, and kept alive by this nervous energy.

In fact, most of the wealth of Western capitalism was not created from necessity, but as a consequence of the discharge of anxiety-generated nervous energy. Being unnatural, capitalist surplus production must be created by irrational forces.

This unnecessary or superfluous capitalist production became a status symbol, which became a booster to the lonely individual's ego, and this increased anxiety which provided more nervous energy for more luxury or status symbols production.

The superfluous also became beautiful.

As a great deal of the capitalist production of the superfluous is the result of an unscrupulous exploitation of the limited resources of our planet, it seems clear that the superfluous, however beautiful it may look, is realised at the expense of what might be essential for future generations.

What is even more pathetic is that many parents justify their unscrupulous pursuit of material wealth in order to impress their children, to leave them this wealth in order to provide them with a better standard of living and higher material independence. These parents, however, also leave their children an overexploited environment, polution, an endangered planet, and increased insecurity and anxiety.

Spending on the superfluous or unnecessary increases the ego's infatuation and its pretentiousness, which increases anxieties. In order to placate these anxieties, more and more people increase their spending on the superfluous or the unnecessary, resulting in the mental disorder, 'spendomania'.

Some experts explain that overspending is a drug which makes people 'high'.

Being irrational, overspending must be a result of restricted mental activity. As I said before, in states of high anxiety we often reach exhilaration or euphoria. It is in these states of exhilaration or euphoria that our mental activity and behaviour become irrational. It is not overspending that makes us euphoric, it is stress-induced euphoria which makes us overspend.

This stress-induced drugged state is best seen in expensive shops and department stores during the sales. People will queue for hours, often in inclement weather, pushing and fighting in order to purchase superfluous and unnecessary goods with credit cards.

It is a well-known fact that these occasions are a haven for pick-pockets, who always take full advantage of the drugged states of these euphoric customers.

The restlessness and agitation in capitalism can also create a general exhaustion, mental confusion and disorientation, loss of memory, 'yuppie flu', or serious psychosomatic diseases and mental disorders.

Curiously enough, these problems also increase with any step towards more individual freedom in communist countries.

Restlessness, agitation and mobility of the lonely individuals with the adolescent middle-class mentality contributed to the development of an important pillar of capitalism: trade.

Many people insist that capitalism can only operate properly in a climate of free individual competition. This is true, as competition increases loneliness, alienation and hostility, therefore increasing anxiety and its nervous energy.

In the capitalism which glorifies competition, success is idolised. Any culture which idolises success must generate fear of failure. This dread of losing amasses such anxiety-created nervous energy that it gives competition an ugly and brutal side.

Competition is in tune with the adolescent either/or mentality, their agonism and the game they fight in search of their egos assertions.

There is no agonistic and agonising competition in the juvenile mentality and its play, nor in the benevolent and tolerant mature mentality.

Capitalism is kept alive and prosperous by the perseverance and tenaciousness typical of reptilian behaviour, which comes into prominence when the efficiencies of the neo-cortex and the limbic system are weakened by the brain's opiates.

It is on this stubborn reptilian perseverance and this obstinate tenaciousness of the selfish and unscrupulous individuals, in a free society, that the economic surplus or economic growth of capitalist economy is built.

Capitalism in the USA acquired a specific driving force which consisted of immigration, or to be more precise, the immigrant's mentality. It was the immigrants that gave American capitalism its accelerated rhythm and speed.

Many immigrants went to America to make a fortune, as quickly as possible, in order to return with it to their country of origin. Many, however, never returned as they became hooked on the stress caused by the acceleration and speed they introduced. Those who returned to their country of origin left behind their beginners' enthusiasm and speed which helped to shape the rhythm of American economy and the American style of life.

The nineteenth century brought a new idea, an economic theory opposing capitalism. The nineteenth century invented socialism.

How did the idea of socialism come about? What kind of mentality invented it, and what kind of mentality tried to both take advantage of it and abuse it?

My impression is that socialism must have been invented by the philanthropic mature mentality.

Profit-motivated industrial and commercial capitalism, practiced by the unscrupulous adolescent middle-class mentality made life a misery for many.

Faced with the needy and miserable, some people develop a mature mentality with its maternal benevolence and compassion. In fact, charitable organisations in industrialised countries started a new vogue in the nineteenth century. These charities were, and still are, mainly organised by women, as confronted with the needy, women acquire maturity much more easily than ego obsessed men. In fact, while their unscrupulous husbands are exploiting those in misery, their wives are often in charge of the charities dealing with their very victims. Words such as sentimentality and sensitivity, depicting feelings, entered Western languages.

It must have been the humanitarian and maternal way of reasoning of the mature mentality, saddened by the misery created by the unscrupulousness of capitalism, that inspired socialist philosophy, ethics, politics and economy.

As I said before, each mentality or mental attitude has its own brain's glandular activity, its own reasoning and logic, its own ideal economic system. Only a maternal mentality, used to deal with children, could have, for instance, invented the socialist motto; 'From everyone according his abilities, to everyone according his needs.'

A charitable organisation can be highly efficient and productive, even more efficient and productive than a capitalist enterprise when it is organised by the voluntary labour of people with a giving mentality. Socialism, in fact, can be very efficient and extremely productive economically, if it is run by volunteers gathered together in small groups. When it is organised and run on a vast scale, however, by the State as a whole, it becomes another story.

The first philosophers and preachers of British ethical socialism, of French utopian socialism and of Italian Christian socialism were all considering socialism in small groups, with limited numbers of people, run as a family by men and women of good will for men and women of good will. This was almost impossible to realise in a big State, particularly in a world dominated by people with an adolescent middle-class exploiting mentality.

Co-operation is much more efficient than destructive competition, is the logic of maturity's reasoning. But, unfortunately, the majority of people belong to the middle-class adolescent mentality, to whom a voluntary co-operation is a sacrifice, an effort which offends their egos. Their egos are only gratified by personal profit, mainly realised through exploitation.

Individuals of the adolescent middle-class mentality soon realised the vast exploiting potential of socialism. It was this human element with its abundance of nervous energy, plus an exploiting mentality, that re-organised socialism into communism.

The difference between socialism and communism is that the former is mainly led and organised by people with a benevolent mature mentality and can only be efficient if all society is composed of those with a mature mentality, while the latter is run and organised by individuals belonging to the adolescent middle-class mentality. In fact, most communist leaders were, and still are, of an opportunistic, exploiting, Machiavellic middle-class mentality. Communist leaders realise equality for the masses, often in misery, but they fight unscrupulously for their own individual priviledges. There is little difference between an American businessman and a Soviet political commissaire: they are both obsessed with self-interest. I am sure that if a successful Western businessman emigrated to a communist country he would soon become a leading member of the communist party, just as if a leading member of a communist party in the East were permitted to leave, he would soon become a successful businessman in the West.

On the other hand, when a political dissident from a communist country emigrates to the West, he might either continue to fight the established order in his chosen new country, or he could develop withdrawal symptoms like drug addicts when on cold turkey. For many dissidents, challenging the communist regime, is exciting, even euphoric, as it boosts the secretion of the extra quantity of brain opiates.

Stalin must have known that communist revolutionaries, as any other revolutionaries, were addicted to the brain opiates. In fact, when he came to power, he imprisoned or killed most of those revolutionaries who had helped communism come to power. He must have realised that most of them would have revolted against him in time, in search of excitement and brain opiates.

Capitalism and communism are competitive because they are both run by elements of the same mentality, unscrupulously and cynically opportunistic, both idealising and idolising crafty cleverness, a result of the shallow and narrow short term way of reasoning.

Communism is inferior to capitalism, however, where economic efficiency is concerned. In order to create equality, communism had to eliminate private property and individual freedom, thus eliminating much anxiety and anxiety generated nervous energy, this essential factor to capitalism and its productivity.

Communism considers itself a revolutionary movement. With its restlessness, agitation and permanent pursuit of the novelty and innovations, and with its permanent tendency to expand, however, capitalism seems to be more revolutionary than communism. By introducing more certainties through static and lasting rules and laws, communism tends towards stagnancy.

The increasing number of aged and those dependent on State assistance, and the vast number of people unable to cope with capitalism and its competition and values, all live in hope that one day humanity might adopt some kind of humanitarian socialism. But this would only work if it was run by the mature mentality element. The mature mentality element, however, can never succeed while the adolescent middle-class mentality dominates world. The only way, therefore, that the mature mentality could come into prominence would be the collapse of the adolescent middle-class culture.

The threat of nuclear anihilation could be the incentive to the adolescent middle-class mentality to grow up and reach maturity. The prolifteration and proliferation of nuclear weaponry and power just might accelerate the arrival of an era of human maturity.

Liberating us from our mind's wishful or pretentious attitudes, a positive fear, such as nuclear anihilation, might bring humanity to a more mature longer term way of reasoning.

Perhaps, however, it is too late. Humanity is becoming more and more intoxicated by the stress-generated opiates, created by the constant potentiality of total annihiliation.

For millions of years our ancestors lived in groups from which evolved the extended family. From the large family the nuclear family evolved, composed of husband, wife and their children. Recently more and more one-parent families are in vogue.

More and more people choose to stay single for ever. After a certain period of the drugged state created by being single, these confirmed bachelors and spinsters prefer to remain in their stress-induced drugged state than to face the reality of married life. In the mind of these single people, the stress-induced drugged state is more exciting than the predictability of a married life.

For a social species, remaining single is selfishness at its maximum, selfishness generated by the brain working under stress and stress-induced opiates.

Individuality and its loneliness brought another uniqueness in nature: suicide.

There is evidence that loneliness stimulates the activity of the hypothalamic–pituitary–adrenal axis of glands. It is known that an excessive activity of these glands can create a state of depression resulting in suicidal behaviour.

There is also evidence that stress caused by loneliness can influence the glandular activity of our brain and the secretion of neurotransmitters. A reduced secretion of the neurotransmitter serotonin, seems to be related to suicidal behaviour.

Individuals belonging to collectivities or cultures which practice individuality are more susceptible to suicidal behaviour than individuals belonging to collectivities or cultures stressing the importance and values of the community. There are also more suicides among single people than the married, among those living in restricted families than among those living in extended families, among people living in a city than among those living in villages, among individuals of the middle-class than the working-class, among people living in more prosperous economies than those living in the Third World. It is also interesting to note that there are more suicides in periods of growing economies than in states of stagnancy or decay.

The cult of individuality developed a new form of love: self-love or selfish love. Loneliness craves being loved.

Self-love is a result of the insecurity and precariousness in which an adolescent mentality's ego exists. The more an ego is in danger, the more self-centred it becomes and the more it loves itself. An ego loves whatever loves it, aleviates its precariousness, or flatters its infatuation.

The adolescent mentality's love exploits. To this exploiting mentality, beauty is whatever can provide it with flattering profit or gain. Flattery, profit or gain are the major gratifications for an insecure ego.

The adolescent mentality's lonely individual brought another novelty in nature: hatred. Hate is only generated by the mind's inflated ego. Only an ego can hate. In fact, the more inflated an ego, the greater the potential of its hate. An ego hates whatever intimidates or threatens its infatuation.

The adolescent mentality's ego brought another uniqueness in nature: passion. Passionate love and passionate hate belong to the adolescent mentality's ego infatuation. The energy that passionate love and passionate hate need is provided for by the nervous energy that the anxiety, which accompanies infatuation, generates.

In its fragility and precariousness, the adolescent inflated ego develops another passion, that of possessions of whatever can please or flatter it. The adolescent inflated ego also develops a passion for the destruction of whatever threatens or offends it.

Passion for possessions inspired another of the mind's inventions: jealousy.

That jealousy is a creation of the mind can be seen by the fact that the energy needed to keep it festering is provided for by the nervous energy supplied by the anxiety, which is generated by the dread of losing of a possession.

The most common source of jealousy is suspicion of a partner's infidelity. The stressful dread of losing ego-flattering fidelity can disharmonise our brain's glandular and mental activities so to create mental disorders of paranoic proportions.

There is much confusion about the idea or definition of love. Perhaps this is because humanity is composed of different mentalities each with its own idea or definition of love, its own conception of togetherness and intimacy, its own favourite kind of relationship, its own idea about sex and sexual relationship.

There are three main human mentalities: the juvenile mentality, or Homo ludens, the adolescent mentality, or Homo credulus, and the mature mentality, or Homo sapiens.

Those with a juvenile or child-like mentality tend to be attracted to people who provide care and protection, such as those with the mature mentality. Feeling protected encourages playfulness and charm.

Those with a mature mentality are usually attracted to the needy, as by exercising their generousity, tenderness and benevolence, they find fulfilment and content. The love of the mature mentality is a maternal love which consists of generousity, tenderness, benevolence, pity and sympathy.

The juvenile and mature mentalities are attracted to each other in a particular way. The juvenile mentality's playfulness and the mature mentality's sense of humour have much in common, they complement each other.

The intelligence and wisdom of maturity is built on the understanding of other people's needs, shortcomings or vulnerabilities. Obviously, there is only one way towards a better understanding of others and that is less self-centredness.

Parents could help their children to mature by owning up to their own failures, their own vulnerabilities and shortcomings. By playing the role of perfection and self-sufficiency, parents alienate their children. Perfection and self-sufficiency diminish intimacy and communication, and without these, there is no understanding or togetherness. Shortcomings, need and vulnerability are major stimulants of communication.

Confronted with the sick or invalids, most people acquire a mature mentality which implies assistance, care or help. Beggers in the street approach the potential donor distorting their faces or bodies in order to inspire maturity, therefore generosity.

The adolescent mentality individual can never establish togetherness or intimacy with anyone. Due to his selfishness and self-love, he is permanently trying to exploit or take advantage of others, and particularly of those who love him.

The prefered targets of the adolescent mentality's exploiting love are the juvenile mentality's innocence and the mature mentality's benevolence. An inflated ego considers these exploitations results of his crafty cleverness. Crafty cleverness seems to be the greatest flatterer of the inflated ego. In the eyes of the inflated ego, cleverness increases with the increase of its treacheries, cheating, lies and hyposcrisy.

Certain individuals with strong adolescent mentalities

are happily able to debase, abuse, torture and even kill old people, beggars, invalids or anyone in need of help. This might be due to the fact that they are irritated by the crippled or elderly as the sight of these wretched people might stimulate maturity, and individuals with the capricious adolescent mentality detest whatever and whoever tries to take their drugged mentality from them. In their strong and stubborn adolescent mentality, caring for others would reduce their drugged state. Most cruelty is committed in the defence of a drugged ego.

Those threatened by these vicious adolescents usually try to placate them by appealing to their kindness or humaneness, or by begging for mercy. This, however, only infuriates them more, increasing their violence.

Ever since the male adolescent mentality imposed itself on humanity, women's maturity has increased. This increase was stimulated by the precariousness and vulnerability in which man placed himself with his infatuations and wishful beliefs. Woman's maternal love felt pity for her adolescent mentality men as they became pathetic in their performance anxiety or stage stress generated by their assumed roles, roles inspired by the wishfulness or pretentiousness of the mind.

Woman continued, and still continues, to be benevolent and charitable with her man, even in bed, when stark naked, he still plays a role. In maturity, pathos and humour fuse into maternal tenderness.

With women's liberation, however, more and more prefer to imitate the adolescent mentality man and assume his attitudes.

With this attitude of women, more and more man/woman relationships are based on mutual exploitation, the exploitation of two self-loves. This often cynical and unscrupulous exploitation forces more and more people towards lonely lives.

This continuous increase in the number of lonely people could be likened to the following experiment. When a fragment of liver and a fragment of skin are broken into their single cells, then placed into an incubator, they will reaggregate in order to form fragments of the organ from which they came from. When the same experiment is repeated with a mixture of cancerous liver and skin cells, the incubation does not produce fragments of the organs from which they came. Individual cancer cells remain separated from each other.

Anxiety carried by lonely individuals brought another uniqueness in nature: obsession with the sex. We are the only species who practices sex in all seasons and at all hours of the day and night.

The adolescent mentality's male ego feels the need to prove its validity whenever it is shaken by reality which, given its pretentiousness, is a permanent possibility. Sexual prowess tends to be the most appealing to an ego built around the idea of masculinity and virility. It is also one of the easiest to achieve as it is possible to develop sexual readiness purely by using our fantasies.

Anxiety-generated nervous arousal provides the energy necessary for sexual seduction and sexual activity.

Conditioned by the adolescent mentality's culture, many women adapt themselves to man's world. They find their best method of survival in being, or pretending to be, what is expected of them. 'Man wants to be pleased in his ego, so, let's please him,' is the motto of many women.

In many cases, man's suplication, or begging for sex, revives women's maternal feeling, therefore, benevolence and generosity. Man will seldom realise, and certainly never admit, how many of his seductions and successes were in reality due to women's pity or charity.

Many women on reaching middle age actually feel pity for their husbands when a sudden increase in their adolescent mentality, due to their threatening middle-age crisis, they decide to leave their wives for much younger women.

Sex with other animals, with small children, or between homosexuals, is usually practiced by people unable to find pleasure in normal sex. Their pleasure comes from stress-induced opiates, generated by the challenge or rebellion against nature or against the established order.

Adulterous sex, especially in Catholic countries, provides a special excitement because of the stress-induced brain opiates provided by the sin. Perhaps, sin, and the cult of sin, was dreamed up to experience that extra pleasure that sinning provides. Some people even experience an additional dose of pleasure when confessing their sin.

There is a frigid, self-confident female element, usually from a socially respectable but perhaps dull background, which only seems to find pleasure by going against the establishment and having intimate relationships with villains, rogues and dangerous criminals.

It is with sex that the difference between anxiety and stress is best illustrated. A moderate range of anxieties creates nervous energy which in turn provides the energy for sexual activities. A high range of anxieties or stress, however, can create sexual impotency. This is particularly evident with students studying for exams, or for actors and actresses just before the opening of a new performance.

The adolescent mentality also developed two other novelties in nature: the tragic and the comic.

In essence there is no difference between a tragedy and a comedy: in both there is a pretentious or conceited ego fallen from its illusions or expectations into the reality of the life.

If we sympathise with a fallen victim because his failure threatens our own illusions, then we will consider this failure a tragedy. To the adolescent mentality tragedy is often related to the 'irony of fate'. The irony of fate seems to belong to the world of faith, to the world of excessive illusions or expectations.

Those who are amused by the failure of a conceited ego, will find it comic. A fully dressed cardinal or a decorated general in uniform, slipping on a banana skin is a definite source of mirth, but the same accident happening to a cripple, blind man or pregnant woman is not funny at all.

Basically we are amused by the fall of those representing pretentiousness, pomposity or conceit, a role or an attitude, because they carry intimidation or threat. Their fall releases our nervous energy.

Each mentality reacts differently to the failure of a pompous person. The adolescent mentality will probably suffer with them or sympathise. The juvenile might laugh or giggle, while the mature mentality might smile benignly, and offer their help.

The urban middle-class mentality enriched its languages. Flowery or euphemistic language became of vital importance to a mentality leaning on roles, poses and assumed personalities, a mentality trying to impress. In fact, most people belonging to this mentality spend a great deal of their lives enduring performance anxiety or stage stress.

It must have been this mentality of poses and masks which invented and perpetuated the theatre.

Because the brain of the urban middle-class is influenced by its reptilian legacy, is perhaps the reason why its language is cooler and more distant than the emotional language, expressions and gesticulations, a result of the brain activity under the influence of the limbic system, or the more economic and succinct language created by the brain under the influence of its neo-cortex.

Affectations, facades, deceptions, ritualism, formalism or mannerism became the life of the urban middle-classes, a life or urbanity. Urbanity became a virtue or a sign of civility or refinement.

To the middle-classes, anything that was not urban was vulgar, in other words anything that was natural. The middle-class mentality considers itself above nature and naturalness.

In his escape into privacy, the middle-class lonely individual became prudish. Prudery influenced dress fashions and nudity became indecent or obscene.

It is interesting to note that in parts of the world or periods of history in which there was no strong middle-class influence, no such word or concept of prudery existed.

To the juvenile mentality, nudity inspires a playful intimacy.

For the mature mentality, indecency only starts where beauty ends. Indecency, however, does not offend maturity as it evokes tenderness.

In the nineteenth century, middle-class prudery reached the limit when it was considered necessary to put skirts on tables and chairs in order to hide the legs!

Possibly in order to placate the anxiety caused by loneliness, the middle-class developed self-discipline, self-control, orderliness, time-tables, punctuality and cleanliness. Cleanliness was more a show of seemliness than the need for hygiene.

In order to feel safer, perhaps, the lonely middle-class individuals also introduced pedantry. The cult of pedantry developed into a passion for detail which before long became an obsession for the particular.

With the rise of the middle-classes the use and passion for mechanical clocks arrived.

What could have inspired the idea of a mechanical clock and the passion for it? What kind of mentality could have started adapting its biological clock to an artificial one?

Only an over-ambitious or pretentious mentality could have disrupted its biological rhythm with a mechanical one more in accordance with the mind's aspirations than with the needs of the body.

The gap between the adaptation to the mind's mechanical clock and the body's biological clock creates tension, anxieties and stress.

The invention of the mechanical clock must have been preceded by a deeper awareness of time and the pressure caused by it.

A deeper awareness of time must have been the result of the brain's activity under a certain range of anxieties. In fact, awareness of time is noticeably reduced in existences without anxieties.

Anxiety and emptiness caused by an individual's loneliness must have increased the awareness and pressure of time. Time seems much less present in the mind when in the company of others.

An increased awareness of time generates tension. Tension creates a sense of duration. In the mind's idea of Paradise there is no tension, there is no duration or time. Paradise implies eternity.

Boredom, another characteristic of lonely individuals, is also intimately related to an increase in the awareness of time. In fact, bordom is mainly caused by an intimidation of time.

Rigid mechanical precision and scrupulous exactitude are very much in tune with our reptilion legacy. It is, perhaps, this legacy which helped the human brain to invent the mechanical clock. The mechanical clock is not at all in tune with the flexibility of the limbic system or the tollerance of the neo-cortex.

Awareness of time became an obsession in which time became a tyrany and its victims robot-slaves blindly serving their tyrant.

Discovering time, the middle-class mentality started exploiting it unscrupulously.

The avid exploitation of time created a sense of urgency: time famine. Overscheduling is becoming more and more of an obsession. Overscheduling gives the impression of exploiting time at its maximal level. This flatters an individual's sense of self-importance, which is a drugged state of existence. Perhaps, it is because of this that people love living under pressure, their diaries filled with appointments they consider important.

This is probably why so many people dread losing time. Lost time is lost importance. To a precious ego, time is precious. 'Time is money,' as the saying goes, which, of course, is true for those who worship money. Many try to save time by rushing.

Increased rushing and overscheduling has led to more and more queueing, waiting and congestions. But, although we are aware of this we still persist in doing it. Perhaps, it is because the frustration of queueing, waiting and congestion increases the stress-induced opiates in our brain.

That awareness of time is related to our minds can be seen from the fact that each mind has its own particular awareness of time which also varies according to time and space for each individual mind.

That the notion or awareness of time is intimately related to each individual mind can also be seen from the fact that when the mind's ego is flattered, times flies. When the individual ego is instead threatened or under pressure, time seems to last for ever. An ego is mostly aware of time when it is desperately awaiting hopeful gratification.

Awareness of time, and the passion for timing, are

reduced to minimal proportions in the juvenile mentality's playfulness and in the mature mentality's serenity.

More and more lonely individuals are becoming intent on a comic pastime, that of trying 'to find themselves', their 'real inner selves', their identities.

Individuals belonging to this mentality can never find their identity because it is merely in their imagination which changes in accordance with the change in the discontent of the mind. Some people rightly call this 'deep inner self' personal identity, rightly, because 'persona' originally meant a mask, an assumed attitude, a performed role. People invent their 'self', then pretend the right to fulfil it.

That this 'deep inner self' is a wishful creation of the individual's mind is evident as it carries much anxiety or stress. Stress-induced opiates, generated by a strong-minded assumed identity, can, in fact, create a drugged state.

This identity game, played by so many lonely adolescent individuals, reminds me of a joke. In a lunatic assylum an inmate is playing Patience. Another inmate approached and pointed out that he was cheating. 'I know,' he smiled, 'but I am so good at it now, I do not even notice.'

The cult of individuality found a powerful ally in the television, as it helps to increase isolation and loneliness. By increasing loneliness, watching television also increases the stress-induced opiates in the brain. In fact, many people spend hours in front of their televisions in drugged states.

Changing channels by simply pressing on an electronic gadget also increases intoxication, giving an illusion of power. In fact, many people spend much of their viewing time changing channels for no reason.

Those who claim that children learn a lot from television, usually selfish adolescent minded parents who can not be bothered to play with or talk to their offspring, ought to know better. Children rarely follow the story, contents or coherence of a cultural program with attention, but the program's special effects. What is more, children also love the power game of changing the channels.

Having missed out on the pleasures of reading or playing communal games, those who spend their childhood glued to television have more difficulty later in learning as their perception of communications is distorted.

The cult of individuality's major aim is individual independence.

In their search for individual independence, many people reach the surrogate of individual independence: individual indifference. With individual indifference loneliness increases.

We are becoming so drugged by our individual indifference that we concentrate most of our energy in defending it, in protecting it against emotionality or understanding.

It seems that the stress caused by our obsessive search for more and more individual independence is placing the human brain more and more under the influence of our reptilian heritage.

Our scientific and technological progress manipulated by the reptilian legacy does not promise a great future.

Courses in Anxiety and Stress

Given the major influence that they play in human life, I think that lessons on anxiety and stress should be introduced in schools and universities.

These courses on anxiety and stress should also be introduced on the shop floors of factories.

These courses should explain the connection between anxiety and the efficiency of our senses and perceptions, the higher the anxiety, the lesser the efficiency. In extreme stress the efficiency of our sense/perception can be reduced to the minimal level, even disappear.

Obviously, the lesser the efficiency of our sense/perception, the lesser is our participation in life.

Due to a significant reduction of the efficiency of their senses and perceptions, excessively self-centred people become isolated from reality. They have great difficulty in recovering from this isolation as their only possible means would be through an improvement of the efficiency of their perceptions of reality. Reduced participation in life can develop into agoraphobia.

All this would not be surprising if one took into consideration that it is in the nature of reptiles to live in hiding and isolation.

High anxiety can also distort the relationship between the senses and perception. We often perceive a threatening person or happening as much more frightening or horrific than it was in reality. Rape victims, or the victims of robberies tend to describe their assailants much stronger and bigger than they really were.

In comparison to the adolescent mentality, the juvenile and mature mentalities have a much keener efficiency of their senses and perceptions. A mature mentality parent hears her or his child moving or crying while a parent of the adolescent mentality might not.

Women are generally more intuitive than men because, due to their higher maturity, their senses and perceptions are more efficient.

In imitating the male adolescent mentality, however, many liberated women have reduced the efficiency of their senses and perceptions and therefore of their intuitive abilities.

Perhaps it is due to the evolution of the complexity of our mind and of its anxieties that our species is so far behind other mammalians as far as the efficiency of our senses is concerned.

These courses should explain that certain fixed ideas or deep rooted beliefs can create a neuronal fixed frame or structure in the brain, providing chronic anxiety. The more rigid the belief, the more rigid is the neuronal fixture in the brain, which limits its glandular and mental activities.

With the mind's fixed frame, firmly embedded in the brain, the synaptic connections between the neurons are less active and less flexible, which inhibits reasoning and memory. Those who dedicate their lives to deep prejudices or fixed ideas, usually those with adolescent mentalities, suffer far more from senile dementia than those with more flexible minds.

Brains dominated by adolescent mentality's frames consume far less oxygen and glucose than brains dominated by juvenile and mature mentalities. Many people spend most of their lives only using approximately 30% of the capacity of their brains.

We are proud of our big brain, but a trivial prejudice or a capricious wishful belief can reduce its activity to pathetic proportions and results. For example, a club or regimental tie, a uniform, a decoration, a hair-cut, or a title can frame the brain, reducing its glandular and mental activities to unhealthy proportions.

These courses should emphasise that with the cult of individuality and individual isolation, which provide stress and stress-related brain opiates, we live a life of drug-addicts.

Many were excited with the discovery of natural opiates in 1973 because of their ability to reduce physical pain.

The secretion of our opiates, however, is not only caused by physical pain but more by the mind's self-induced suffering. This is what brings on an addiction to our own opiates.

These courses should explain that these opiates can also affect our brain's mental activity. If narcotic drugs or alcohol can reduce our sense/perception and our reasoning, or alter our consciousness, then we should expect our brain opiates to be able to do likewise.

As I explained, in reality our brain is composed of three brains: the new brain or the neo-cortex, the mammalian brain or the limbic system, and the reptilian or old brain that we inherited from our reptilian ancestors.

Under the influence of stress and stress-related brain opiates the first brain to be affected is the last comer in evolution, the new brain, the brain where our broader and deeper reasoning and reflexive awareness take place.

The first sign of the influence of stress-related natural opiates over the new brain can be seen in the reduced efficiency and accuracy of our language which centre lies on the left hemisphere of our neo-cortex. (In fact, autistic children who seem to have an excessive secretion of brain opiates have difficulty in acquiring a language.)

Under stronger stress, the brain opiates start affecting our mammalian brain which lies under the new brain and which evolved before the neo-cortex. Shaken in its efficiency by the brain opiates it affects our emotional life and our interpersonal relations. The mammalian brain deals with social bonding, family life, maternal care and protection, safety in togetherness and gregariousness.

When our limbic brain's efficiency is thrown by stress opiates our mental activity and behaviour become dominated by our oldest brain, the brain we inherited from our reptilian ancestors. The main characteristics of the mental activity and behaviour dominated by our reptilian legacy are emergency impulsiveness, automatism, instant gratification, violence, cruelty, nastiness, deviousness, extreme selfishness and self-centredness, here and now reasoning, and unscrupulous self-preservation.

In fact, the human mind might have had its inspiration for ideas of evil, the devil and infernal forces in the reptilian legacy. After all, it was a reptile which tempted Eve to commit original sin.

Many mental disorders are generated by an excessive influence of the reptilian brain. The most attrocious crimes in history were committed by those in a state of euphoria, a state in which mental activity and behaviour are dominated by the primitive reptilian brain.

There is evidence that during stress, metabolic activity and blood flow increase in two specific areas of the brain. This happens in the regions of the temporal poles of the neo-cortex where, most probably, wishful beliefs and prejudices, which create and perpetuate stress, take place, or where the stressful experience is perceived. During stress metabolic activity and blood flow also increase in the parts of the old brain which deals with emergencies.

Many experts advise people under stress to reason themselves out of their problems, to pull themselves together. These experts clearly do not realise that the stress which accompanies these problems usually unbalances the efficiency of the new brain, the only brain capable of reasoning us out of any problems.

The experts also insist that the main difficulty of those under stress is that they bottle up their feelings instead of airing them. They claim that these wretched people have no-one to talk to.
Under the influence of the reptilian legacy people seldom listen to others' miseries or problems. Perhaps this is why they do not realise that anyone would listen to theirs.

It is obvious that we are addicted to our own opiates by the fact that we tend to create unnecessary problems, that we like to magnify difficulties, that we enjoy risking our lives indulging in dangerous sports, that we are attracted and excited by uncertainties, even that we seem to revel in suffering.
When the brain opiates are not sufficient to give us a kick, then we start using and abusing of narcotic drugs and alcohol.
Most people who drink or abuse narcotic drugs know the peril they run. But may be it is living with peril itself that gives them the extra 'high'.

These courses should explain that, due to self-induced drug-addiction, we are a species which can be manipulated or seduced with ease. Our historical past offers many examples of blind obedience to the most obvious absurdities and the most irrational religions or ideologies. This blind and servile obedience can only be explained by stress-addiction.

These courses should emphasise that there are no biological differences between the brains of different races. The only difference between races is the difference in the use of their brain, ruled by the mind's frames mainly consisting of prejudices. In a community of racial discrimination, the brains of both the discriminator and the discriminated are under the influence of the reptilian legacy.

In communities dominated by racial prejudices there are relatively more people with mental disorders than in communities with racial tolerance.

These courses should explain that national prejudices can create similar anxieties, therefore similar reasoning and behaviour of the people of that nation. It is, in fact, the similarity of anxieties which mainly contribute to a nation and its characteristics.

Crafty governments often manipulate collective anxieties in order to be able to manipulate the reasoning and attitudes of their citizens. Many political leaders try to make their people insensitive to serious local problems by reducing the efficiency of their senses and perceptions and creating national anxiety by provoking international tensions or a foreign threat.

Providing similar anxieties, similar environmental conditions can provide a similarity of reasoning and behaviour.

Experiencing similar anxieties, marginal groups in all parts of the world reason and behave in a similar way.

Experiencing similar degrees of anxiety, strong believers, be they Christian fundamentalists in the USA or Muslim fundamentalists in the Lebanon will all show a similar reasoning and behaviour, similar intolerance and aggression. The most blood-thirsty wars have always been religious wars.

The teachers of these courses should re-write national histories. Everyone tends to see their national past through rose tinted glasses, but the new editions should point out stupidities and errors as well as victories and successes.

Humbleness improves the efficiency of the senses and perceptions, and helps people to reach a broader and deeper way of reasoning.

Beliefs in national superiority create national hooligans of all kinds.

Common Market countries would have more in common if their national histories showed their mistakes and sillinesses. Europe could be united for ever by merely explaining the absurdities of the last two world wars.

These courses should explain that Western knowledge serves cleverness, not intelligence. Cleverness concentrates on the efficiency of methods and means, because its only aim is here and now exploitation and profiteering. For cleverness, the end justifies the means.

Operating on the here and now basis, cleverness implies unpredictability, therefore apprehension and tension, anxiety and stress. Operating on a longer and broader perspective, intelligence implies a lesser apprehension and tension, lesser anxiety or stress.

In the hands of the middle-class mentality, knowledge increases arrogance and aggression. The Nazi crimes were prepared and executed by very knowledgable people, with highly qualified scientific methods. The XIX Century provided more learning and knowledge in the West than any other century, but it also produced the arrogant and aggressive beliefs, the highly efficient and extremely clever exploitation of colonies, and more revolutions and wars than any previous century.

With the juvenile mentality knowledge enriches play and playfulness. With the mature mentality knowledge increases humbleness and understanding.

Many people spend most of their lives leaning on wishful beliefs. The mind's wishfulness is a result of the tendency of instability towards lesser instability.

Each wishful belief and each degree of a wishful belief carries its own doubt, its own precariousness, and every doubt or precariousness carries its own anxiety or stress.

Each anxiety and each stress carries its own activity of the hypothalamus, its own secretion of neurotransmitters and hormones, and each of these secretions carries a certain tension or malaise in the body.

These physical changes produced by anxiety or stress, increase the mind's discontent which tends to find lesser discontent through the mind's expansion. This increases the mind's complexity, therefore, its instability. This creates more anxiety or more stress. Any increase in complexity creates more problems than it solves.

The natural end of the evolution of the continuous expansion of the mind, therefore, is mental insanity. In fact, the constant increase in human restlessness and agitation, in crime and violence, in envy and intolerance, in the consumption of narcotic drugs, barbiturates and alcohol, and in mutual callous indifference, shows a persistent increase in mental instability.

That we are steadily drifting towards mental instability is also evident from the fact that we are more and more attracted by people with an obvious distortion in their senses and minds, particularly in the field of art and literature. What is more, we are sometimes so seduced by the work of these mentally unstable artists or authors to the point of excitement or ecstasy, even calling them geniuses.

History is filled with examples of those seduced by mentally insane political or military leaders. In fact, mental insanity creates the masses generating mass euphoria and thus mass irrationality.

It is a curious phenomenon that the masses are created by an excess of the cult of individuality. In his stress-related addiction the lonely individual finds his final escape in belonging to the masses dominated by mental insanity.

A lonely individual increases his drugged state when part of the masses, as he feels more protected and more confident in his wishful fantasies. This feeling of increased confidence is what makes the masses so dangerously aggressive and destructive.

These courses should explain that humanity also risks new epidemics due to the progressive increase in the stress-induced immunodefficiency. We can see how a group like male homosexuals, which is under an above average stress, has a higher susceptibility to opportunistic infections and AIDS than the rest of the population. In fact, the spread of AIDS and the increase in opportunistic infections among male homosexuals coincides with the restlessness, agitation and stress produced by the gay liberation movements.

As I mentioned before, male homosexuality mainly consists of the mind's attitude of challenge to natural order. Any new freedom obtained by a challenge implies more challenge, more stress and more health hazards. Challenge, which is only a human phenomenon, is an important contributor to stress-addiction.

These courses should also explain that with the increase of stress and stress-addiction, impotency and sterility increase.

For a long time humanity has hoped that the mind and its creativity would provide the solution for human discontent and suffering. This illusion is drifting more and more towards disillusion.

These courses should explain that we should not be surprised by the increasing ugliness, confusion and malaise created by the mind's creativity in art, philosophy, politics and economy.

The negative side of illusions is that they generate natural opiates which shake the realistic reasoning of our brain. With realistic reasoning one could easily discover that the mind with its wishfulness can not provide any practical solution. The mind is the result of an escape, and an escape carries emptiness, and emptiness cannot but create illusions, or hopes, and more emptiness. Escape is a defeat.

Those who flatter humanity and glorify the human brain, promising a great future, are basically cruel. It is cruel because it is pushing drugs on drug-addicts. It is cruel because it is guiding the blind towards a precipice.

Many insist, and in a dramatic way, that humanity is in a tragic situation.

I think that humanity is not so much in a tragic but a comic situation. Hoping to find the solution for their difficulties in wishful speculations or pleasing fantasies is pretentious, and pretentiousness is the source of ridicule.

Our addiction to hopes, however, can be explained by hopes' ability to create stress and by the ability of stress to generate brain opiates.

Being abstractions, hopes have no positive values. When they sometimes are realised, they soon disappear leaving the mind with its inherent emptiness and discontent.

Perhaps, humanity's complaint of being in a crisis, a crisis beyond repair, is the mind's way of having an extra secretion of the brain opiates, yet another clever discovery of stress-addiction.

These courses should explain that we can only reach a broader way of reasoning through humbleness, as only through humbleness can we reduce stress-addiction, because humbleness reduces pretentiousness. This is the only way to slow down the evolution of humanity towards mental insanity.

These courses should explain that the evolution of our

mind towards more complexity, more instability and more insanity cannot be stopped, and even less reversed. This truth could in fact help humanity, particularly the ruling middle-class adolescent mentality, to find humbleness. Through humbleness this mentality could either reach the playful juvenile mentality or acquire the sense of humour of the mature mentality. In this way perhaps we could slow down the expansion of the mind towards more complexity. In this way perhaps we could develop a new belonging in order to reduce stress. Humour carries tenderness and tenderness goes hand in hand with togetherness.

We take ourselves overseriously which is not serious, we consider ourselves important and indispensible which makes us laughable.

These courses should explain that laughing at oneself prevents one becoming laughable.

In reality, our main problem is our obsessive dread of becoming ridiculous. Self-ridicule, on which a sense of humour is based, can prevent anyone from becoming ridiculous.

By the same author:

'HUMOUR THERAPY in Cancer, Psychosomatic Diseases, Mental Disorders, Crime, Interpersonal and Sexual Relationships.'
  '*Your theories make good sense – and the stories you use to illustrate the theories are delightful.*' Norman Cousins who recovered from cancer curing himself with humour therapy.
ISBN 0 9510525 0 0
Pbk. Price: £5.00

'SPY IN THE VATICAN 1941–45'.
'*War: opera buffa*' ... '*Mr. Bokun tells us these stories with the irony and compassion they deserve. His style is inobtrusively brillant.*' The New York Times.
'*A slavic version of Catch-22*'. Washington Post.
'*One of the most vivid and authentic contemporary pictures yet published in English of Rome during this period.*' Publishers Weekly.
'*A sensitive account of life in a foreign capital in wartime. He depicts with wry vivacity a half-world of spies and counterspies.*' The Economist.
ISBN 0 9510525 2 7
Pbk. Price: £5.00